A Clinician's Guide to Progressive Supranuclear Palsy

A Clinician's Guide to Progressive Supranuclear Palsy

Lawrence I. Golbe

Rutgers University Press

New Brunswick, Camden, and Newark, New Jersey, and London

Library of Congress Cataloging-in-Publication Data

Names: Golbe, Lawrence I., author.
Title: A clinician's guide to progressive supranuclear palsy / Lawrence I.
  Golbe.
Description: New Brunswick, New Jersey : Rutgers University Press, 2018. |
  Includes bibliographical references.
Identifiers: LCCN 2018009740 | ISBN 9780813565965 (pbk. : alk. paper)
Subjects: | MESH: Supranuclear Palsy, Progressive
Classification: LCC RC388 | NLM WL 358.5 | DDC 616.8/36—dc23
LC record available at https://lccn.loc.gov/2018009740

A British Cataloging-in-Publication record for this book is available from
the British Library.

♾ The paper used in this publication meets the requirements of the
American National Standard for Information Sciences—Permanence of
Paper for Printed Library Materials, ANSI Z39.48-1992.

www.rutgersuniversitypress.org

Manufactured in the United States of America

CONTENTS

PREFACE

Progressive supranuclear palsy (PSP) first appeared in the medical literature only in 1963. Until then, it was typically misdiagnosed as Parkinson disease (PD), which it outwardly resembles to a variable degree. As a vestige of that era, PSP is still informally classified as a "Parkinson-plus syndrome" or an "atypical parkinsonian syndrome."

PSP shares with PD slowness and paucity of movement, muscle rigidity, and impaired balance. These cardinal features arise from the 2 diseases' mutual involvement of the substantia nigra, a nucleus in the midbrain that uses dopamine as its neurotransmitter. But PSP produces far more profound involvement of the frontal cortex, basal ganglia, brainstem, and spinal cord than does PD. While PD does in most cases cause some degree of frontal dementia, balance loss, eye movement difficulty, dysarthria, dysphagia, and incontinence, in PSP, these are more important relative to the cardinal "parkinsonian" features, and they appear earlier in the disease course.

But what makes PSP one of neurology's thorniest problems is its poor response to levodopa or any other treatment. Patients with PD before the levodopa era survived an average of 8 years from onset, but that figure has now more doubled. For PSP, average survival remains a dismal 7.4 years, about a year less than that for the classic form of PSP, called PSP–Richardson syndrome.

The burden of PSP for patient and family is exacerbated by its frustration for health professionals. Conspiring to produce that frustration is apathy as part of the neurological syndrome, lack of a specific diagnostic test, and mysterious causation. Its low incidence causes a "why bother?" problem, and its advanced average onset age of 63 years causes a "you've got to die of something" problem. This book hopes to counter those professional prejudices and frustrations as much as it hopes to inform patient care.

This technical level here is for neither laypersons nor movement disorder neurological subspecialists. Rather, this book addresses the needs of general neurologists, primary care physicians, nurse practitioners, physician assistants, hospital nurses, psychiatrists, psychologists, ophthalmologists, optometrists, oto-laryngologists, speech and swallowing therapists, physiatrists, physical thera-pists, urologists, and radiologists. It is not for neuropathologists or laboratory scientists, although they may benefit from the general clinical overview here.

The volume is organized to be read cover to cover but is also usable as a reference. At every turn, it discusses research opportunities and challenges, serv-ing as a resource and inspiration for clinical investigators designing projects.

I provide references only selectively. They are intended more as suggestions for further reading than as meticulous documentation of my statements. It's easy enough to visit Medline for an exhaustive, current list of references.

In my experience, health professionals confronted with a patient with PSP are most interested in 3 basic questions: (1) How is PSP diagnosed? (2) How do I know when a newly reported symptom is part of PSP, as opposed to part of an unrelated illness? and (3) How is PSP managed? This book will emphasize these 3 issues.

Research against PSP is finally bringing this disease into the modern era. There are now validated diagnostic criteria and a validated clinical rating scale. Genetic marker risk factors have been identified, and sequencing is pro-ceeding. Multiple animal models have been created. Many details of molecular pathogenesis have been worked out even if we do not yet understand their importance relative to one another in actually causing cell death. We have multiple imaging procedures, and diagnostic markers in blood and cerebro-spinal fluid are nearly here. There have been a handful of large, double-blind treatment trials. Such activity started long ago for many disorders, but PSP has now caught up. So clinicians have fewer reasons for frustration and patients have fewer reasons for despair. I hope this book makes life better for both.

A Clinician's Guide to
Progressive Supranuclear Palsy

History 1

It seems remarkable that a disease so vividly recognizable was not clearly described in the literature until 1963. In that year, J. Clifford Richardson (1909–1986), a neuropsychiatrist at Toronto General Hospital and Sunnybrook Military Hospital, reported clinical and pathological findings in 7 patients at the annual meeting of the American Neurological Association (ANA) in Atlantic City, New Jersey (Pearce, 2007). The paper appeared in *Transactions of the ANA* later that year (Richardson et al, 1963). The second author was John C. Steele, Richardson's resident at the time. The third was Jerzy Olszewski (1913–1964), pronounced "ol-SHEF-skee," a neuropathologist at the Banting Institute at the University of Toronto. He published a pathologically oriented description of the same cases in the *Journal of Neuropathology and Experimental Neurology* in the same year (Olszewski et al, 1963).

A more detailed analysis of the clinical and pathological data under the authorship of Steele, Richardson, and Olszewski appeared the following year, 1964, in the leading American clinical neurology journal of the time, *Archives of Neurology* (Steele et al, 1964). The eponym "Steele-Richardson-Olszewski syndrome" or, less commonly, "Steele syndrome" was used for many years but now has nearly disappeared in the literature, particularly in the United States. However, now that various clinical phenotypes characterized by progressive supranuclear palsy (PSP) pathology have been described, the term *Richardson syndrome* has been assigned to the classic clinical form of PSP as described in the 1963 to 1964 publications.

Dr. Steele continued to publish on PSP and on the related disorder, lytico-bodig (Guamanian ALS-parkinsonism-dementia complex). Now in his 80s, he remains an energetic and articulate ambassador in the fight against PSP and an inspiration for young researchers.

Richardson's first patient was a personal friend, a 52-year-old business executive, who first consulted him in 1955 for difficulties with cognition, vision, and balance. By 1962, his autopsy and those of 6 other patients with similar clinical pictures became available.

Sporadic reports in the literature before 1963 are incomplete but highly suggestive, and some were cited by Steele, Richardson, and Olszewski. In the 1880s at the Hôpital de la Salpêtrière in Paris, Jean-Martin Charcot (1825–1893), often considered the founder of modern neurology, published and lectured on patients with atypical parkinsonian conditions, including a retrocollic form that could have been PSP. Overall, 13 published cases of what could have been PSP were published before 1963. Six of them included autopsies that in retrospect are compatible with PSP.

Dickens provided a tantalizing account of what could have been PSP in his 1857 novel, *The Lazy Tour of Two Idle Apprentices*:

> A chilled, slow, earthy, fixed old man. A cadaverous man of measured speech. An old man who seemed as unable to wink, as if his eyelids had been nailed to his forehead. An old man whose eyes—two spots of fire—had no more motion that [*sic*] if they had been connected with the back of his skull by screws driven through it, and riveted and bolted outside, among his grey hair.
>
> He had come in and shut the door, and he now sat down. He did not bend himself to sit, as other people do, but seemed to sink bolt upright, as if in water, until the chair stopped him. (Larner, 2002)

There are multiple reasons for the tardy appearance of a clinicopathologic description of PSP. Parkinson disease received its clinical description in 1817, its description of Lewy bodies in 1912, and the localization of its major pathology to the substantia nigra by Tretiakoff in 1919. Alzheimer described clinical and pathologic features of "presenile dementia" in 1907. The various phenotypes of multiple-system atrophy, which even in total are less common than PSP, were described earlier, the cerebellar form by Déjerine and Thomas in 1900, the dysautonomic form by Shy and Drager in 1960, and the parkinsonian form by van der Eecken et al in 1960.

One reason for PSP's late arrival is that its pathology is nearly identical to that of postencephalitic parkinsonism, at least by the histopathologic methods available before tau immunostains arrived in the 1980s. Since the encephalitis lethargica epidemic of 1917 to 1928, a neuropathologist encountering such a case would likely have concluded that the clinical encephalitic illness was mild or misdiagnosed. Clinicians encountering a patient with PSP would have diagnosed either Parkinson disease with unusual "rigidity" of the extraocular muscles and neck extensors or "arteriosclerotic parkinsonism," described by Critchley in 1929. The senior academic neurologists, whose reactions to Richardson's 1963 ANA presentation were published along with the formal description, remarked that they had not seen this syndrome in their own referral practices. But they did not dispute the validity of the observations and, upon returning to their clinics, began to notice such patients.

This is a specialized example of a "scientific revolution" as described in 1962 by Thomas S. Kuhn in *The Structure of Scientific Revolutions*. Kuhn's seminal observation, now taken for granted, is that false scientific models persist despite the slow accumulation of contrary evidence. The old model bends to admit successive small changes, in this case by incorporating the concept of "atypical parkinsonism." Only when the contrary evidence becomes overwhelming does the old model collapse, in this case by recognizing the existence of a new disease. Kuhn coined the term *paradigm shift* to describe this phenomenon.

Shortly before the 1963 to 1964 publications, Olszewski showed a patient and the slides of the autopsied cases to Asao Hirano, a neuropathologist at Montefiore Hospital in New York who had described the neuropathology of lytico-bodig in 1961. Hirano, like many others since, was struck by the clinical and pathologic similarities and suggested that a common cause might be found, perhaps infectious or toxic. Dr. Steele, who spent much of his career on Guam as a general neurologist, worked tirelessly to find such a common thread, to motivate and organize specialists toward that goal and to facilitate their visiting Guam. The most recent theory holds that the cause may be dietary exposure to beta-methyl amino L-alanine, an excitotoxin produced by cyanobacterial commensals in tree roots, then concentrated in fruits, then in the animals that consume them, and finally in people consuming the animals.

More recently, Guadeloupean tauopathy was discovered as another geographically isolated tau-based neurodegenerative disorder with clinical similarities to PSP in many cases. Evidence exists for a causal role of annonacin, a mitochondrial toxin in certain tropical fruits. Although the evidence of dietary causes for both the Guamanian and Guadeloupean disorders remains incomplete, it does provide plausibility for a dietary contribution to the cause of PSP itself.

The following table shows some of the notable achievements in basic and clinical research against PSP since the seminal papers of Steele, Richardson and Olszewski.

1973	Tellez-Nagel et al	Differentiation of neurofibrillary tangles (NFTs) of PSP from those of Alzheimer disease
1986	Pollock et al	NFTs found to be principally hyperphosphorylated tau
1988	Golbe et al	First prevalence study and diagnostic criteria for PSP
1995	de Yébenes et al	First and still largest autosomal-dominant PSP family
1996	Conrad et al	A dinucleotide repeat polymorphism called A0 in *MAPT* (the tau gene) is slightly overrepresented in PSP
1996	Litvan et al Hauw et al	Clinical and pathological criteria for PSP delineated through analysis of a large autopsy series of parkinsonian disorders
1996	Golbe et al	First demonstration of lesser educational attainment as a risk factor for PSP
1997	Arai, et al	First report of cerebrospinal fluid (CSF) tau findings in PSP
1999	Chambers et al	Tau with 4 microtubule binding sites predominates in neurofibrillary tangles of PSP, differentiating it from Alzheimer disease, where NFTs have equal shares of 3- and 4-repeat tau
1999	Schrag et al	First community-based PSP prevalence study
1999	Caparros-Lefebvre et al	Description of cluster of PSP-like illness on Guadeloupe; association with consumption of *Annona* species, which contain the mitochondrial toxin annonacin
1999	Baker et al	Report that the A0 allelic locus is part of a larger haplotype, H1
1999	Albers et al	Demonstration that mitochondrial dysfunction is critical in PSP
2000	Lewis et al	First tau mouse, a knock-in of human MAPT gene with P301L mutation
2001	Wittmann et al	First tau fruit fly (*Drosophila*)
2003	Kraemer et al	First tau roundworm (*Caenorhabditis elegans*)
2003	Kato et al	Description of the hummingbird sign on magnetic resonance imaging (MRI), caused by isolated midbrain atrophy
2004	Champy et al	Annonacin in rats reproduces many features of PSP
2004	Kwok et al	Observation of increased tau expression by the H1 haplotype
2005	Williams et al	Observation of 2 separate clinical phenotypes sharing nearly identical PSP pathology: Richardson syndrome and PSP-parkinsonism
2007	Golbe et al	Publication of a validated PSP clinical rating scale
2007	Williams et al	Description of pure akinesia with gait freezing as a third PSP phenotype

(continued)

2008	Stamelou et al	Coenzyme Q-10 found to have modest symptomatic efficacy in PSP in a double-blind trial
2009	Bensimon et al	First large, double-blind treatment trial, the Natural History and Neuroprotection in Parkinson Plus Syndromes (NNIPPS) study, shows riluzole ineffective
2009	Frost et al	Demonstration of spread of tau aggregates between neurons and induced fibrillization of target cell tau, similar to prion disorders
2011	Höglinger et al	Whole-genome search using single-nucleotide polymorphisms shows 4 previously unsuspected risk loci: MOBP, EIF2AK3, STX6, and a second MAPT locus
2011	Evidente et al	Autopsies of neurologically asymptomatic cases show the lifetime incidence of PSP pathology to be 15 times that suggested by clinically based incidence surveys
2013	Clavaguera et al	Demonstration that tau from humans with PSP can template its specific pathology onto mouse tau after intracerebral injection, supporting the "prion hypothesis" for PSP
2014	Boxer et al	Davunetide, a neurotrophic factor, shows no neuroprotective efficacy in a large, double-blind trial
2014	Tolosa et al	Tideglusib, a GSK-3β inhibitor (to reduce tau phosphorylation), shows no neuroprotective efficacy in a large, double-blind study using the PSP Rating Scale as the primary outcome measure
2014	Höglinger et al	MRI volumetry from the tideglusib study shows evidence of slowing of MRI atrophy in whole brain, whole cerebrum, parietal lobe, and occipital lobe
2014	Li et al	First demonstration of abnormal methylation of genome in PSP
2015	—	Anti-tau antibodies BMS-986168 and C2N-8E12 enter clinical trials
2015	Caparros-Lefebvre et al	Report of the first PSP geographical or temporal cluster, in Wattrelos, France, a site of marked environmental contamination by metals
2017	Passamonti et al	Positron emission tomography using ^{18}F-AV-1451 found to distinguish PSP from Alzheimer disease (but not from controls)
2018	Rojas et al	Ratio of neurofilament light chain to phosphorylated tau in CSF found to predict progression of PSP over the following year
2018	Sanchez-Contreras et al	SLCO1A2 and DUSP10 identified as new PSP genetic susceptibility loci via single-nucleotide polymorphism data

Descriptive Epidemiology 2

JUST HOW RARE IS PSP?

Patients with progressive supranuclear palsy (PSP) and their families may feel "orphaned" because PSP is rare and most physicians know little or nothing about it. It may be helpful to point out to such patients that PSP is approximately as common as amyotrophic lateral sclerosis. The prevalence of PSP has been formally measured using community-based ascertainment in only 4 places: London and Newcastle in the United Kingdom; Rochester, Minnesota; and Yonago, Japan. Each study gained access to the medical records of a community and sifted out those that suggested PSP (Bower et al, 1997; Kawashima et al, 2004; Nath et al, 2001; Schrag et al, 1999). Then, the researchers evaluated those candidates further to ascertain the positive cases using uniform diagnostic criteria. Each of the 4 studies found about 4 times as many PSP cases in this way as had already been diagnosed by a physician to have the condition.

The 4 studies each found between 5 and 6 cases per 100,000 population, while the number already diagnosed as PSP in each of the populations was 1 to 2 per 100,000. Two other studies that assessed the prevalence of PSP from existing medical records also arrived at figures between 1 and 2 per 100,000 (Golbe et al, 1988). This means that in the United States, with a total population of 320 million, there are 3600 to 7200 people with an existing diagnosis of PSP. The total with PSP would be 16,000 to 19,200 if only they could be evaluated by a professional familiar with PSP. (Hence this book!)

Incidence is the number of new cases of a disease over a defined period, typically 1 year. For PSP, the figure is 1 or 2 per 100,000 population. Multiplied over an 80-year life span yields 80 to 160 per 100,000. Stated more simply, about 1 in 1000 people develops clinically diagnosable PSP sometime during life. However, a 2014 study from a large retirement community in Arizona found PSP pathology in 5% of autopsies in people who were neurologically normal just before death (Dugger et al, 2014). If the mild PSP pathology in fact is a precursor of the more severe pathology seen in symptomatic individuals, this finding suggests that the clinical diagnosis represents a small tip of a much larger lifetime incidence iceberg.

Assuming worldwide uniformity of PSP incidence and duration of survival (not a safe assumption for countries with poor medical care of the elderly), the total number of living patients worldwide with clinically symptomatic and diagnosable PSP would be between 362,000 and 433,000.

Prevalence is the number of existing, living cases regardless of recency of diagnosis. Table 2.1 shows the prevalence of PSP in the context of other neurodegenerative and/or parkinsonian disorders. The figures use as their "denominator" the overall population, not the elderly population. These figures will surely rise as the population ages, barring developments in disease prevention or cure. Further advances in general medical care may prolong survival of disabled patients, raising the disease prevalence. The apparent prevalence will rise as physicians become more adept at recognizing early or atypical PSP.

TABLE 2.1 Approximate PSP prevalence compared to that of other neurodegenerative diseases

	Approximate prevalence per 100,000 overall population
Corticobasal degeneration	<1
Multiple-system atrophy	4
PSP	**5**
Amyotrophic lateral sclerosis	6
Behavioral variant frontotemporal dementia	20
Dementia with Lewy bodies	100
Parkinson disease	150
Alzheimer disease	1600

Note: The data were collected using various methods and populations.

ONSET AGE

The onset age of PSP cannot be calculated with certainty. It depends on the age structure of the underlying population, and most reports do not adjust the raw average. (The onset age of PSP in a retirement community such as Sun City, Arizona, will be higher than in a typical population.) Furthermore, when the onset starts with a symptom other than a fall, it occurs so gradually that assigning a specific date is arbitrary. That said, the mean onset age has been reported as 59 to 65 years. The standard deviation of onset age, typically about 7 years, is less than in, for example, Parkinson disease (PD), where it is 11 years. (About two-thirds of all cases fall within 1 standard deviation of the mean.) This suggests that the range of causative factors of PSP is more narrow than that for PD and therefore may be easier to understand and to address with disease-modifying therapy. Or so one can hope.

SURVIVAL

Duration of survival in PSP varies across studies, with the typical figure between 7 and 7.5 years after the onset of symptoms (Jecmenica-Lukic et al, 2014; Arena et al, 2016; Bang et al, 2016; Ghosh et al, 2013; Golbe et al, 2007). For PSP–Richardson syndrome (RS), which accounts for about half of all PSP, the median figure is somewhat lower, about 6 years, while for PSP-parkinsonism, which accounts for about 25%, it is about 9 years. Many studies have attempted to identify factors influencing survival in PSP that may be of benefit in counseling patients and families. A 2017 review and meta-analysis (Glasmacher et al, 2017) found that the only acceptably consistent predictors, aside from the PSP-RS phenotype itself, were early dysphagia, early cognitive symptoms, and early falls. It is not clear, however, whether these 3 operated statistically independently of one another or of the PSP-RS phenotype, the definition of which includes those features as early or prominent components of the syndrome. Figure 2.1 shows survival curves stratified by PSP Rating Scale (PSPRS) score. It will assist in advising patients after administering the PSPRS.

Most studies of prognostic factors in PSP have only assessed the statistical association of longer survival (or time to milestones) with the presence of the candidate factor. But as part of my own effort to validate the PSPRS, I assessed the time to reach important disability milestones and death based on the total PSPRS score. My thinking was that the patient asks, "How long 'till I can't

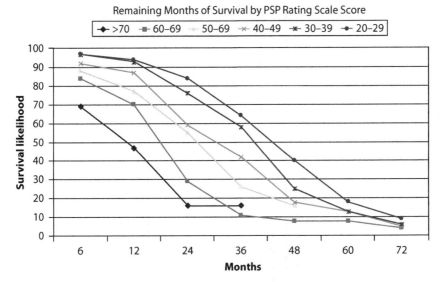

FIGURE 2.1 An approximate guide to remaining months of survival in patients with PSP, stratified by PSP Rating Scale score. This used patients at all stages and with all phenotypes but only after they had progressed to the point of fulfilling the National Institute of Neurological Disorders and Stroke—Society for Progressive Supranuclear Palsy criteria, which were designed for Richardson syndrome. The 95% confidence intervals are considerable and are given in Table 2.3.

walk?" and not "What features of my illness correlate with time to inability to walk?"

To that end, Table 2.2 shows the percentage likelihood of retaining the ability to walk independently at each of a number of timepoints, stratified by PSPRS score. The outcome variable used PSPRS item 26, entitled "gait," and the milestone was attaining a score of 4, defined as, "Unable to walk, even with walker; may be able to transfer." The table shows the percentage likelihood of failing to reach that score, along with its 95% confidence interval. For example, patients at the time of PSP diagnosis typically have a PSPRS score in the 30s. Their likelihood of still being able to walk, at least with some type of assistance, is 72% at 12 months, 42% at 24 months, and 16% at 36 months. It is important to draw the patient's attention to the confidence intervals and to explain their meaning.

Table 2.3 is similar but uses death as the milestone. For the patient in the example above, the likelihood of remaining alive is 93% at 12 months, 58% at 36 months, and 6% at 72 months. Again, the 95% confidence intervals are

TABLE 2.2 Percentages (95% CI) of patients retaining at least some gait ability (ie, PSPRS item 26 < 4) at the given intervals

PSPRS score	Percentage still walking independently (95% CI)					
	6 months	12 months	24 months	36 months	48 months	60 months
20–29	93.1 (88.0–98.5)	76.4 (67.5–86.5)	48.8 (37.2–64.1)	22.7 (12.3–41.9)	13.6 (5.7–32.7)	9.1 (3.0–27.1)
30–39	92.3 (86.7–98.4)	72.4 (62.7–83.7)	41.8 (30.1–58.1)	15.9 (7.9–32.0)	a	a
40–49	90.2 (83.1–97.9)	51.7 (40.0–66.9)	21.7 (11.8–40.0)	6.5 (1.8–23.5)	a	a
50–59	64.7 (51.5–81.4)	39.1 (26.2–58.5)	11.1 (4.0–30.4)	a	a	a
>60	42.9 (25.4–72.2)	21.4 (9.9–46.3)	a	a	a	a

aNo patients reached these timepoints with gait score less than 4.

TABLE 2.3 Survival estimates and 95% CI for patients with total PSPRS scores in the specified ranges. Survival times are calculated as the interval between initial entry into the specified score interval and death.

PSPRS score	Subsequent survival percentage (95% CI)						
	6 months	12 months	24 months	36 months	48 months	60 months	72 months
20–29	97.1 (91.9–100)	94.2 (86.8–100)	83.8 (71.8–97.7)	64.1 (48.7–84.5)	40.1 (25.4–63.1)	18.0 (8.1–40.2)	9.0 (2.5–32.0)
30–39	96.4 (91.7–100)	92.6 (86.0–99.7)	76.4 (65.7–88.8)	57.7 (45.3–73.6)	25.3 (15.1–42.3)	12.6 (5.6–28.5)	6.3 (1.8–22.6)
40–49	91.5 (85.2–98.1)	86.9 (79.4–95.2)	58.9 (47.9–72.5)	41.9 (31.0–56.6)	17.9 (10.2–31.5)	13.0 (6.5–26.2)	5.2 (1.5–18.5)
50–59	88.0 (80.6–96.0)	76.9 (67.4–87.6)	54.9 (44.0–68.6)	26.0 (16.8–40.2)	16.2 (8.7–30.2)	a	a
60–69	83.7 (74.1–94.4)	70.2 (58.5–84.3)	28.5 (17.8–45.4)	11.4 (4.7–27.6)	7.6[b] (2.5–22.8)	7.6[b] (2.5–22.8)	3.8 (0.9–16.6)
>70	69.2 (54.9–87.2)	47.4 (33.0–68.0)	16.4[c] (7.5–30.4)	16.4[c] (7.5–30.4)	a	a	a

[a]Not estimable because there were no survivors.

[b,c]These are the same because there were no observed deaths between the 2 successive timepoints.

important, and I expect to publish a refinement of these prognostic data in late 2018 that narrows the confidence intervals and conditions the outcomes on other clinical variables. The data in Table 2.3 appear in simplified, graphic form in Figure 2.1.

Analytical Epidemiology 3

ENVIRONMENTAL AND LIFESTYLE RISK FACTORS

A poorly studied aspect of progressive supranuclear palsy (PSP) is the nongenetic component of its etiology. There have been only 4 published studies. The first 3 are relatively small (Golbe et al, 1988; Golbe et al, 1996; Vidal et al, 2009) as such studies go, with 50, 91, and 79 cases with PSP, respectively, and the fourth used 284 newly ascertained cases (Litvan et al, 2016). Three of the 4, including the largest, found that lesser educational attainment was more common among people with PSP than among controls. The 2 smaller studies gave odds ratios of 0.35 and 0.38, respectively. The largest gave an odds ratio of 0.59. Only one of the studies assessed dietary factors, finding that relative to controls, patients with PSP had consumed less fruit and more meat or poultry.

The question about educational attainment was included in the PSP studies because it was previously known that lesser education is associated with Alzheimer disease. A popular hypothesis to explain this relies on the notion of "synaptic reserve," which holds that education promotes the development of cerebral synapses. This provides a degree of redundancy to brain function so that if and when a degenerative process comes along decades later, an educated person is less likely to suffer a deficit and therefore more likely to be included in a control group than in an Alzheimer disease group. It would be reasonable to extend this hypothesis to explain the same observation PSP.

Another plausible explanation for the observation of lesser educational attainment in PSP is that people with blue-collar jobs tend to suffer more exposure to toxins, whether at work or in residential areas close to industry. None of the case-control studies has been able to associate a specific occupation or toxin exposure to PSP. The oft-confirmed association of pesticides and herbicides with Parkinson disease (PD) does not exist for PSP, according to the few available studies.

Interestingly, all 4 studies agreed that the well-confirmed association of PD with nonsmoking was absent in PSP. The same is true for the association of lesser atherosclerotic risk with PD. The explanation for the first is unknown. The explanation for the second may be that PSP does not share PD's tendency to hypotension. The association of PD with higher melanoma risk and with low risk of most other cancers has not been assessed in PSP. Coffee consumption is known to be less in PD than in controls, but this relationship does not exist in PSP, again for unclear reasons.

PSP is a sporadic disorder except for the few, usually small familial occurrences described in the chapter on genetics. PSP does not even appear to have the racial differences documented in PD, although most studies show that men are affected a bit more often than women. Nor has there been any evidence for any temporal trend or clustering in PSP incidence. We should, however, not forget the informal observation of many of the leading neurologists of the early 1960s that upon learning of the series of Steele et al, they could recall no such patients of their own. But in the ensuing years, they did start to make the diagnosis with some regularity. Unfortunately, no one has studied this observation properly.

A GEOGRAPHICAL CLUSTER

The first known cluster of typical PSP was reported by my colleagues and me in 2015 (Caparros-Lefebvre et al, 2015). It was discovered and clinically characterized by Dr. Dominique Caparros-Lefebvre. In a group of suburban towns centered on Wattrelos and Leers in northern France, there have appeared 100 cases of PSP from 2005 to 2017. This is 12.4 times the expected incidence based on formal population studies in the United Kingdom, United States, and Japan, the only places where such studies have been performed.

The patients in the cluster displayed only 2 features atypical of PSP elsewhere. One was that the fraction of cluster patients with Richardson syndrome, 33%, was far lower than the fraction in the original description of Williams et al (2005), 53%, but close to the 24% seen in a more recent series that, like the analysis of the cluster, considered the full range of other PSP phenotypes (Respondek et al, 2014). The other atypical feature of the cluster was an older onset age than typical, 74.3 years vs the mid-60s for most series. This is despite a population age distribution for the Wattrelos area that is typical for Western countries where the series of sporadic PSP were gathered. Thirteen of the 100 have come to autopsy, which showed typical PSP in all with no more concomitant pathology than expected in this age group. A wide range of clinical features occurred in the 100 patients, as expected for any such series of patients with PSP.

At first glance, the most obvious candidate as a cause of the cluster is a genetic founder effect. However, none of the 100 patients knew of a relative with PSP, and only 12 knew of a relative with a diagnosis of Alzheimer or Parkinson disease. Furthermore, 7 of the patients were of Algerian descent, with little or no genealogical connection to the northern European majority.

The most likely explanation of the cluster is a toxin related to the area's industrial past. A factory that processed chromate and phosphate ores was near the center of the area where the 100 cases lived. It dumped its spent ore in large piles next to the factory. The factory itself was demolished in the 1980s, but the piles remain. While only 2 of the 100 patients actually worked in the factory, the spent ore contaminates much of the residential area, a situation exacerbated by periodic floods and by use of dredgings from an adjacent river as landfill for construction of roads and athletic fields. The metals in the ore piles may also have found their way into private garden plots used for raising vegetables for home use. Also in the area for much of the 20th century were textile dying and leather tanning plants, both of which use products from the chromate plant. In progress are studies of the cluster's molecular genetics, toxic exposures, residential and occupational histories and dietary habits, and renewed attention to metals in case–control risk factor surveys outside of the cluster's area. This cluster may provide a valuable and perhaps pivotal clue to the cause of all PSP.

Clinical Rating Scales 4

Despite the elusiveness of any proven, specific intervention for progressive supra-nuclear palsy (PSP), clinicians need a tool by which to track the state of the illness quantitatively in individual patients. Physicians should assess any symptomatic benefit of dopaminergics, coenzyme Q-10, or various nonpharmacologic therapies and discontinue them in cases where their benefit is absent, transient, or exceeded by adverse effects. Another use of a rating scale is to provide formal clinical treatment trials with a quantitative "outcome measure" or "clinical end point" that is sensitive to change and that reflects the level of disability in daily activities. Just as important is the prognostic information that a rate of progression provides for patients and families, who find some comfort in the knowledge that the deficits are progressing no faster than expected. If the progression is slower, they are encouraged and may find more satisfaction in their remaining years, and if faster, they can use that information to plan for future care or financial arrangements. A quantitative rating scale can also have diagnostic value where documented absence of disease progression over a year's time should prompt suspicion of a nondegenerative process such as a dysimmune state, hydrocephalus, or "vascular PSP."

Two scales specific to PSP have been published: the PSP Rating Scale (PSPRS) and the PSP Quality-of-Life Scale (PSP-QoL). Also available is a scale for use in both PSP and multiple-system atrophy (MSA), the Natural History and Neuro-protection in Parkinson Plus Syndromes–Parkinson Plus Scale (NNIPPS-PPS).

THE PSP RATING SCALE

First, a disclaimer: I am the author of the PSPRS. Published in 2007 with the help of statistician Pamela Ohman-Strickland, PhD, it comprises 28 items scored either 0-2 or 0-4, with 0 the best possible total and 100 the worst. The first 7 items, with 28 of the 100 possible points, concern daily activities as ascertained by interview. The other sections are Mental (4 items, 16 points), Bulbar (2 items, 8 points), Supranuclear Ocular Motor (4 items, 16 points), Limb (6 items, 16 points), and Gait/Midline (5 items, 20 points). The PSPRS appears as Table 4.1.

The average patient has reached a score of about 20 at the time a diagnosis of PSP becomes possible using the National Institute of Neurological Disorders and Stroke and Society for Progressive Supranuclear Palsy (NINDS-SPSP) criteria, and most clinical trials have reported average baseline PSPRS scores of 30 or 35. The score progresses an average of 11.4 points per year through the disease course until the end stage.

At a score of about 75, the total ceases to progress: a "ceiling effect." One reason is that some of the items' maximum score definitions do not accommodate the worst possible state. An example is the patient whose unaided falling frequency at home scores the maximum of 4 because the frequency would be at least 30 times per month without the walker. His deficit may subsequently progress to an inability to use a walker, but the score of 4 still applies. A second reason for the "ceiling effect" is that some of the 28 scale items never exceed zero for some patients, even in the final months. Frequent examples are irritability, tremor, dystonia, and apraxia.

The PSPRS takes 10 to 15 minutes to administer, making it feasible for use in a busy clinic where follow-up visits for patients with complex conditions are scheduled for 30 minutes. The published version of the scale includes tips on administering the scale, and Table 4.1 shows an expanded version. It is advisable to have the tips readily available for reference during the administration of the scale. Several exam items require skill and experience in the neurological exam. Assessing cognitive function, eye movement, limb and neck rigidity, apraxia, and postural stability are the most important examples. However, these can be certainly learned by nurses and other professionals. (I like to brag that my senior research nurse practitioner, Debbie Caputo, is the second-most experienced person in the world in the use of the PSPRS.) The only apparatus required for the PSPRS is a cup of water with which to test swallowing. Also highly advisable is a clear path for gait testing and a wall as a backup for examiner and patient during the pull test (item 27).

The most important general principle to keep in mind when applying the PSPRS is to put the patient's safety first. If an assessment presents some risk for

TABLE 4.1 The PSP Rating Scale

	Section and item	Rating definitions	Instructions and tips
Activities of daily living (ADLs) by history			
1	Withdrawal	0 None	Ask caregiver.
		1 Follows conversation in a group; may respond spontaneously but rarely initiates	Use your own observation. Rate relative to baseline personality.
		2 Rarely or never follows conversation in a group	Consider lack of conversation due to dementia or bradyphrenia as "withdrawal."
			If patient never has opportunity to interact with people other than the caregiver, use direct observation of patient's behavior in exam room.
2	Aggressiveness/ Irritability	0 None	Ask caregiver about frequent loss of temper, shouting.
		1 Increased over baseline but not interfering with family interactions	Relative to baseline personality.
		2 Interfering with family interactions	Ask if shouts or loses temper easily.
			If resists caregiver's care but this does not risk patient's well-being, score a 1. If it does risk well-being, score a 2.
3	Dysphagia (while eating)	0 Normal: no difficulty with full range of food textures	This concerns solid foods only.
		1 Tough foods must be cut up into small pieces	Ignore difficulty related to overloading mouth.
		2 Requires soft solid diet	If the caregiver feels that solids must be cut smaller than typical for patient's size, score a 1.
		3 Requires pureed or liquid diet	
		4 Tube feeding required for some or all feeding	If certain foods like bread crusts or leafy vegetables must be avoided, but meats are OK, score a 2.
			Ignore the issue of patient's manual ability to cut food.

(continued)

TABLE 4.1 The PSP Rating Scale (*continued*)

	Section and item	Rating definitions	Instructions and tips
4	Using knife and fork, buttoning, washing hands and face	0 Normal 1 Somewhat slow but no help required 2 Extremely slow or occasional help needed 3 Considerable help needed but can do some things along 4 Requires total assistance	Rate the worst of the 3 tasks. If difficulty is related to downgaze, score as if it were purely motor. If patient can do buttoning and washing and use a fork but not a knife, score a 3.
5	Falls (average frequency if unaided)	0 None or <1 per year 1 < 1 per month; gait may otherwise be normal 2 < 1 per week to 1 per month 3 < 1 per day to 1 per week 4 At least 1 per day	Can ask patient or caregiver to estimate. Average frequency if attempted to walk unaided except for using walls and furniture. Assume no access to walking aids. Ignore near-falls.
6	Urinary incontinence	0 None or a few drops less than daily 1 A few drops staining clothes daily 2 Large amounts but only when asleep; no pad required during day 3 Occasional large amounts in daytime; pad required 4 Consistent; requiring diaper, pad, or catheter awake and asleep	Ignore excuse of poor ambulation. If daytime pad used as precaution but no recent wetting, score a 3. Define "a few drops" as staining underwear only. If patient uses a pad "as a precaution" during the day, score a 3.
7	Sleep difficulty	0 Neither 1° nor 2° insomnia 1 Either 1° or 2°; averages at least 5 hours per night 2 Both 1° and 2°; averages at least 5 hours per night 3 Either 1° or 2°; averages <5 hours 4 Both 1° and 2°; averages <5 hours	1°: Trouble falling asleep. 2°: Trouble staying asleep (ignore bathroom trips with prompt return to sleep). Ask caregiver about number of hours of sleep. OK to rely on subjective reports. Ignore daytime sleep.

(*continued*)

TABLE 4.1 The PSP Rating Scale (*continued*)

	Section and item	Rating definitions	Instructions and tips
Mental			
8	Disorientation	0 Clearly absent	Ask year, month, date, day, season, hospital, floor, city.
		1 Equivocal or minimal	
		2 Clearly present but not interfering with ADLs	Estimate or ask if problem dictates extra care from caregiver regarding ADLs.
		3 Interfering mildly with ADLs	
		4 Interfering markedly with ADLs	
9	Bradyphrenia	0 Clearly absent	Observe delay for patient to answer easy questions.
		1 Equivocal or minimal	
		2 Clearly present but not interfering with ADLs	Estimate or ask if problem dictates extra care from caregiver regarding ADLs.
		3 Interfering mildly with ADLs	If delayed responses prompt the caregiver to answer for the patient or limit your ability to interview the patient, score at least a 3.
		4 Interfering markedly with ADLs	
10	Emotional incontinence	0 Clearly absent	If none displayed, ask caregiver if patient laughs or cries when others usually do not.
		1 Equivocal or minimal	
		2 Clearly present but not interfering with ADLs	Count conversational interaction as an ADL.
		3 Interfering mildly with ADLs	If there is a history of inappropriate laughing or crying but none at the time of the examination, score a 1 or 2, depending on its frequency.
		4 Interfering markedly with ADLs	
			If the conversation has to pause because of laughing or crying (even if by history), score a 4.
11	Grasping/ imitative/utilizing behavior	0 Clearly absent	Observe grasping of examiner, chair.
		1 Equivocal or minimal	
		2 Clearly present but not interfering with ADLs	Ask caregiver if grasping interferes with feeding, dressing.

(*continued*)

TABLE 4.1 The PSP Rating Scale (*continued*)

	Section and item	Rating definitions	Instructions and tips
		3 Interfering mildly with ADLs 4 Interfering markedly with ADLs	If none is displayed spontaneously (eg, grabbing your coat or arm, or the wheelchair arm), ask patient to rest hands on thighs, palms up. Hold your hands 5 to 10 cm above his or hers and say nothing. If he or she grabs them, rate a 3. If he or she imitates your actions during the exam, rate a 2. If this test is normal, look for applause sign. If claps at least 4 times, rate a 1.
Bulbar			
12	Dysarthria	0 None 1 Minimal; all or nearly all words easily comprehensible to examiner 2 Definite; moderate; most words comprehensible 3 Severe; may be fluent but most words incomprehensible 4 Mute or a few poorly comprehensible words	Ignore palilalia and dysphonia. "Comprehensible" means to examiner, not caregiver. If generally silent but can be coaxed to speak a few words, score a 4, no matter how clear those words may be.
13	Dysphagia	0 None 1 Fluid pools in mouth or pharynx, or swallows slowly but no choking/coughing 2 Occasionally coughs to clear fluid; no frank aspiration	Give 30 to 50 cc of water in a cup, if safe. Do not use a straw. If patient or caregiver insists on a straw, score a 3. If patient finishes the cup without coughing, allow a few seconds more to observe.

(*continued*)

TABLE 4.1 The PSP Rating Scale (*continued*)

Section and item		Rating definitions	Instructions and tips
		3 Frequently coughs to clear fluid; may aspirate slightly; may expectorate frequently rather than swallow secretions	Do not give water if secretions are audible with breathing, if there is a history of frequent aspiration, or if caregiver is apprehensive. In that case, score a 3.
		4 Requires suctioning, PEG, or tracheostomy	One cough scores a 2; multiple coughs scores a 3.
Ocular motor			
14	Voluntary upward saccades	0 Not slow or hypometric; 86% to 100% of normal amplitude	Command the patient to "look up," "look down," "look right," "look left."
		1 Slow or hypometric; 86% to 100% of normal amplitude	For each, start from primary gaze, not the extreme opposite gaze.
		2 51% to 85% of normal amplitude	Do not have patient follow a moving target or direct the gaze to a specific target. However, use a target for primary gaze.
		3 16% to 50% of normal amplitude	
		4 15% of normal amplitude or less	If improves with repetition, use the initial (ie, worst) result.
			For patients who fixate on your face, move away from the patient's primary gaze before testing.
15	Voluntary downward saccades	0 Not slow or hypometric; 86% to 100% of normal amplitude	If you can observe motion rather than just the starting and ending positions, it is "slow."
		1 Slow or hypometric; 86% to 100% of normal amplitude	If a corrective saccade is needed or if the motion is jerky, it is "hypometric."
		2 51% to 85% of normal amplitude	May hold lids to observe downward saccades.
		3 16% to 50% of normal amplitude	Normal range of gaze is 50° in each direction.
		4 15% of normal amplitude or less	Ignore square-wave jerks and other intrusions.

(*continued*)

TABLE 4.1 The PSP Rating Scale (*continued*)

	Section and item	Rating definitions	Instructions and tips
16	Voluntary horizontal saccades	0 Not slow or hypometric; 86% to 100% of normal amplitude 1 Slow or hypometric; 86% to 100% of normal amplitude 2 51% to 85% of normal amplitude 3 16% to 50% of normal amplitude 4 15% of normal amplitude or less	If saccadic speed downward from the up to the primary position is worse than from primary to the down position, consider that "slow" for the purpose of supporting a score of 1.
17	Eyelid dysfunction	0 None 1 Blink rate decreased to <15 per minute 2 Mild inhibition of opening or closing or mild blepharospasm; no visual disability 3 Moderate apraxia or lid opening or blepharospasm causing partial visual disability 4 Functional blindness because of involuntary lid closure	Observe patient in repose. Then have patient open/close lids quickly on command. Recruitment of frontalis muscle scores at least a 2. Isolated difficulty closing lids on command scores at least a 2. If patient keeps lids closed for several seconds at a time, score a 3.

Limbs

	Section and item	Rating definitions	Instructions and tips
18	Limb rigidity	0 Absent 1 Slight or detectable only on activation 2 Definitely abnormal but full range of motion possible 3 Only partial range of motion possible 4 Little or no passive motion possible	Score the worst of the 4 limbs. If apraxia limits relaxation, do not count as rigidity. Count flexion contracture in advanced patients as dystonia, not rigidity. "Activation" means contralateral rapid alternating movement (fist opening or heel tapping). (*continued*)

TABLE 4.1 The PSP Rating Scale (*continued*)

	Section and item	Rating definitions	Instructions and tips
19	Limb dystonia	0 Absent	Rate the worst of the 4.
		1 Subtle or present only when activated by other movement	Ignore neck and face.
			If no dystonia apparent on observation, have patient activate dystonia in this way:
		2 Obvious but not continuous	Hold hands out with eyes closed, palms down. Rate a finger extension or other sustained movement as 1.
		3 Continuous but not disabling	
		4 Continuous and disabling	Tap contralateral fingers or heel.
			Score the worst of the 4 limbs.
			Dystonia in PSP is usually asymmetric.
20	Finger tapping	0 Normal (>14 taps in 5 seconds with maximal amplitude)	Score the worse side.
			Provide example, but stop and rate patient tapping alone.
		1 6 to 14 taps in 5 seconds or moderate loss of amplitude	Have patient hold hand in range of his or her vision.
		2 < 6 taps in 5 seconds or severe loss of amplitude	If abnormal, encourage patient and score the best performance.
21	Toe tapping	Normal (>14 taps in 5 seconds with maximal amplitude)	Score the worse side.
			Provide example and sit far enough from patient to allow his or her range of gaze to see your foot.
		1 6 to 14 taps in 5 seconds or moderate loss of amplitude	
		2 < 6 taps in 5 seconds or severe loss of amplitude	If abnormal, encourage patient and score the best performance.
22	Apraxia of hand movement	0 Absent	If asymmetric, score worse side.
		1 Present, not impairing most functions	Test for ideomotor apraxia.
		2 Impairing most functions	Two tasks with each hand (eg, salute, throw ball, hitchhike, V-for-victory, wave good-bye).
			Apraxic impairment should be evident on casual observation to score a 2. If it is evident only with testing, score a 1.

(*continued*)

TABLE 4.1 The PSP Rating Scale (*continued*)

	Section and item	Rating definitions	Instructions and tips
23	Tremor in any part	0 Absent	If tremor is not otherwise apparent, observe sustention and the finger-to-nose task.
		1 Present, not impairing most functions	
		2 Impairing most functions	Rate the worse side.
			If you clearly see tremor at times during the exam but not during this task, score a 1.
Gait/midline			
24	Neck rigidity or dystonia	0 Absent	Rate the resistance to passive anteroposterior rotation.
		1 Slight or detectable only when activated by other movement	You can ask patient to actively facilitate the passive movement.
		2 Definitely abnormal, but full range of motion (ROM) possible	Ignore spontaneous posture (kyphosis, dystonic rotation, retrocollis).
		3 Only partial ROM possible	If absent, attempt activation by opening/closing both fists.
		4 Little or no passive notion possible	If there is no resistance over some of the range of movement but musculoskeletal resistance thereafter, score a 0.
25	Arising from chair	0 Normal	Use an armless chair.
		1 Slow but arises on first attempt	Be ready to catch patient falling to front or back by putting yourself in front of patient with one hand ready to support neck from behind.
		2 Requires >1 attempt but arises without using hands	
		3 Requires hands	If the patient must use hands, do not allow hands to contact the back of the chair—only the seat.
		4 Unable to arise without assistance	
			If you don't have an armless chair, do not allow patient to push off the chair arms in arising—only the seat.

(*continued*)

TABLE 4.1 The PSP Rating Scale (*continued*)

	Section and item	Rating definitions	Instructions and tips
			Allow patient to reposition forward on the chair, but score at least a 2. Make an exception for short legs.
			If cane/walker needed to arise, score a 4.
			If can arise unassisted but falls forward, score a 4.
26	Gait	0 Normal	Have patient walk at least 15 feet if safe.
		1 Slightly wide based or irregular or slight pulsion on turns	Include at least 1 pivot if safe.
		2 Must walk slowly or occasionally use walls or helper, especially on turns	Tell the patient in advance where to pivot.
		3 Must use assistance all or almost all the time	If patient can walk on a line with minimal difficulty but must use multiple careful steps to pivot, score a 2.
		4 Unable to walk, even with walker; may be able to transfer	If must use walls/furniture to get across the exam room, score a 3.
			If must use a walker or cane, score a 3.
27	Postural stability (on backward pull)	0 Normal; shifts neither foot or 1 foot	Instruct patient to take a step with 1 foot and to try to keep the other foot planted.
		1 Must shift each foot at least once but recovers unaided	If can remain standing unassisted:
		2 Shifts feet and must be caught by examiner	• Explain test • Demonstrate single backward step
		3 Unable to shift feet; must be caught but can stand still alone	• Pull backward by shoulders • Move your hands to a catching position
		4 Tends to fall without a pull; requires assistance to stand still	Have a wall or exam table 1 to 2 meters behind you.
			Pull should be hard enough to make a normal adult take 1 step back to retain balance.
			If this would be unsafe or the result is readily predictable, can score without testing.

(*continued*)

TABLE 4.1 The PSP Rating Scale (*continued*)

	Section and item	Rating definitions	Instructions and tips
28	Sitting down (without using hands)	0 Normal 1 Slightly stiff or awkward 2 Easily positions self before chair, but descent into chair is uncontrolled 3 Has difficulty finding chair behind him or her and descent is uncontrolled 4 Unable to test because of severe postural instability	Have patient approach chair from 3 to 4 steps away with hands on chest. OK to use device to approach chair but not to assist in descent. May not touch the chair with hands but may touch it with legs before sitting. Keep one of your hands close to patient's back to prevent his or her missing the seat or landing too hard.

the patient, estimate the score based on other observations or reports. For example, if the patient or family report that drinking thin liquids always causes coughing and that a thickening agent has been recommended, do not test swallowing with water (item 13). Rather, assign a score of 3 ("Frequently coughs to clear fluid; may aspirate slightly; may expectorate frequently rather than swallow secretions"). Another example is a large patient with obvious balance difficulty, where the result of the pull test (item 27) should be estimated using observation of the gait. This is especially important for smaller examiners, as the procedure for that item requires the examiner to stand behind the patient while applying the pull and to catch him or her if necessary. *Primum non nocere.* To that medical maxim, we should add *etiam te ipsum non nocere* ("also, don't hurt yourself").

The validity of the PSPRS arises from several sources. The original publication used interrater reliability, factor analysis, and the ability of the scale to track progression of the disease longitudinally and to predict the complete loss of gait and overall survival. The score was found to progress 11.4 points per year, with no important departure from this figure at any observed phases of the disease course or at any relevant points on the scale. Since then, several multicenter studies using the PSPRS in placebo groups over a period of a year have corroborated this consistent rate of progression (Apetauerova et al, 2016; Boxer et al, 2014; Leclair-Visonneau et al, 2016; Nuebling et al, 2016; Stamelou, et al, 2008; Tolosa et al, 2014). This helps explain the decision of some drug companies developing tau-based neuroprotective treatment for Alzheimer disease (AD)

TABLE 4.2 Sample size calculation using the PSPRS as the primary outcome measure in a placebo-controlled treatment trial

% change in PSPRS	20	25	30	40	50
Number required per treatment arm	309	198	138	78	51

to first test their product in PSP: the PSPRS is more consistent across studies than the best available clinical scales in AD.

An assessment by Maria Stamelou and colleagues (2016) compared 10 clinical scales used in 2 recent PSP treatment trials to calculate the sample sizes needed for 1-year, placebo-controlled PSP treatment trials using those scales as the primary outcome measure. They found that to detect a 50% treatment effect, the PSPRS would require only 52 patients per study arm, the best performance among those scales for which an adequate sample was available. Next best was the Schwab-England Activities of Daily Living Scale (SEADL), which required 70 patients per arm, and the Clinical Global Impression of Disease Severity (CGIDS), requiring 81 patients per arm. Table 4.2 shows the sample sizes required to demonstrate the given effect size using only the PSPRS score.

The 2 trials providing data for these calculations had a combined dropout rate of 26%. Therefore, the sample sizes above should be divided by 0.74 to calculate the number of patients to be enrolled. An interesting and unexpected observation of this study was that the placebo response rate in PSP was only 10%, while in Parkinson disease, it is typically 30%. This is only a preliminary observation, as the 2 diseases were not assessed in the same trial or using identical methods. However, the observation does encourage researchers that their trials would not be spoiled by a high placebo response rate in PSP despite the observation that the frontal cognitive loss in PSP often increases suggestibility.

The validity of the PSPRS is further supported by its scores' moderate correlation with older, accepted measures used in neurodegenerative disease research. These include the SEADL, the Clinical Global Impression of Change (CGI-c), the Clinical Global Impression of Disease Severity (CGIds), and the Repeatable Battery for the Assessment of Neuropsychological Status (RBANS). The correlation coefficient for these ranges from 0.33 for the RBANS to 0.44 for the CGIds, each with statistically significant 95% confidence intervals (CIs). The change in the PSPRS also correlates to a statistically significant degree with magnetic resonance imaging (MRI) measures of progression in brain atrophy, with the best correlation for midbrain volume, with a correlation coefficient of −.31, followed by whole-brain volume (−.25) (Whitwell et al, 2012). Such morphometric measures of progression of brain atrophy by routine MRI are now the most important secondary outcome measure in neuroprotective trials in PSP.

POTENTIAL WEAKNESSES OF THE PSPRS

As the diagnosis of PSP is not made until an average of 3 years after onset, data on the performance of the PSPRS before that point are sparse. At the other end of the scale, most patients encounter a ceiling effect, where the score typically progresses to about 75 and no further despite ongoing survival, which at that point is typically for a year or less. This is discussed above.

Obvious weaknesses with any clinically based scale are the subjectivity and variability, and in this the PSPRS is no exception. Minimizing these requires close adherence to the scoring tips provided and adherence to a standard method for the examiner that will not change across patients or over time. The PSPRS items where this is perhaps most important are the 4 items in the mental exam and in the assessments of saccadic amplitude and velocity.

HOW MUCH CHANGE IN THE PSPRS IS CLINICALLY MEANINGFUL?

When designing clinical treatment trials, an important question is the size of a clinically meaningful change in the primary outcome measure. In other words, what degree of expected benefit would justify initiating treatment with the agent in question (assuming that any adverse effects are tolerable)? For symptomatic treatments, the "benefit" is the difference between the active drug group and the placebo group with regard to the change from the untreated baseline PSPRS score. For neuroprotective treatments, "benefit" means the difference in the PSPRS rate of change over the course of the study, typically 12 months, between placebo and active drug groups. Even if a statistically significant "benefit" occurs, does its magnitude merit actual use of the treatment in practice?

To answer this question, Sarah Hewer and colleagues mined data from the placebo group of a large PSP treatment trial where 2 of the outcome measures were the PSPRS and the Clinical Global Impression of Change (CGI-c) scale. The latter is a 7-point scale where the middle (fourth) value is "no change relative to baseline" and the 6 flanking points are "marked," "moderate," and "mild" worsening or improvement. The authors assumed that the difference between any 2 adjacent points of the CGI-c to be the minimal observable clinically significant change. They found that over the 12 months of the study, 1 "point" on the CGI-c correlated with an average progression of 5.7 points on the PSPRS (95% CI, 4.83–6.51, $P < .001$). This is almost exactly equivalent to 6 months' progression for the average patient and means that a symptomatic treatment that returns a patient to his or her status from 6 months earlier would be noticeable—and, presumably, appreciated.

THE UNIFIED PARKINSON'S DISEASE RATING SCALE

The UPDRS, familiar to all movement disorder specialists, comprises 4 sections: cognitive/behavioral status, daily activities, motor examination, and complications of treatment. Only part 3, the motor exam, has been used in publications on PSP. Several important features of PSP, such as gaze palsy/saccadic defects, dementia, behavioral changes, sleep problems, dysphagia, and apraxia, are not addressed by that part of the UPDRS. Tremor, which is emphasized in the UPDRS, is rarely much of an issue in PSP. The only items that track the disease course well are bradykinesia and gait. In its favor, UPDRS motor section shows good consistency in PSP (Cubo et al, 2000).

THE FRONTAL ASSESSMENT BATTERY

This brief scale tracks 1 domain of cognitive progression in PSP. It measures conceptualization, mental flexibility, motor programming, sensitivity to interference, inhibitory control, and environmental autonomy. Each of the 6 items is graded on a 4-point scale. Many patients with moderate or advanced PSP have motor difficulty that may affect their performance on the manual tasks in the Frontal Assessment Battery (FAB). Nevertheless, the FAB has diagnostic utility in that it discriminates between PSP and both multiple-system atrophy and Parkinson disease, where there is less of a frontal deficit. It requires much less training than the PSPRS or the UPDRS motor section (Dubois et al, 2000).

MEASURING QUALITY OF LIFE IN PSP

Regulatory agencies—and, more important, patients and families—assign great value to the ability of a prospective treatment to influence quality of daily life. Understandably, they find this more relevant than the results of the neurological examination. The PSP–Quality of Life (PSP-QoL) has been developed by Anette Schrag and colleagues (2006). It correlates well with the PSPRS but includes many areas not addressed in that scale's Daily Activities section. It comprises 45 items, each on a 5-point scale, along with a graphical analog scale on which the patient is asked, "Please indicate how satisfied you feel overall with your life at the moment by putting a cross on the line between 0 and 100." The PSP-QoL meets stringent validity criteria and is an important secondary outcome measure in most clinical trials in PSP. However, its length, requiring

TABLE 4.3 The Health-Related Quality of Life Questionnaire for Patients with PSP (PSP-QoL)

Having a health problem can affect a person's quality of life in many different ways. To help us understand how your illness affects your life, we would like to know which of the following problems you have experienced and how problematic each has been. If the problem does not apply to you, please note why. If someone helps you to fill in the questionnaire, please make sure the answers reflect your own answers. Should you and your helper disagree on the most correct answer, this could be noted at the end. Please note that this list includes many problems which you may never experience.

There are no right or wrong answers. Please think about how you have been feeling during the past 4 weeks. Then check the box for the answer that fits your feelings best.

In the last 4 weeks, have you:	No problem	Slight problem	Moderate problem	Marked problem	Extreme problem	Not applicable
Had difficulty moving?	☐	☐	☐	☐	☐	☐
Had difficulty walking?	☐	☐	☐	☐	☐	☐
Had difficulty climbing stairs?	☐	☐	☐	☐	☐	☐
Had difficulty turning in bed?	☐	☐	☐	☐	☐	☐
Had falls?	☐	☐	☐	☐	☐	☐
Had difficulty moving your eyes?	☐	☐	☐	☐	☐	☐
Had difficulty opening your eyelids?	☐	☐	☐	☐	☐	☐
Had difficulty eating?	☐	☐	☐	☐	☐	☐
Had difficulty swallowing?	☐	☐	☐	☐	☐	☐
Had drooling of saliva?	☐	☐	☐	☐	☐	☐
Had problems communicating?	☐	☐	☐	☐	☐	☐
Had difficulty with your writing?	☐	☐	☐	☐	☐	☐
Had difficulty grooming, washing, or dressing yourself?	☐	☐	☐	☐	☐	☐
Had difficulty using the toilet on your own?	☐	☐	☐	☐	☐	☐
Had difficulty holding urine?	☐	☐	☐	☐	☐	☐
Had difficulty reading?	☐	☐	☐	☐	☐	☐
Had difficulty doing your hobbies, such as playing chess or a musical instrument?	☐	☐	☐	☐	☐	☐
Had problems doing things around the house, such as housework or do-it-yourself projects?	☐	☐	☐	☐	☐	☐
Had difficulty enjoying sports, including gardening or walking?	☐	☐	☐	☐	☐	☐
Had difficulty going out to see a play or movie?	☐	☐	☐	☐	☐	☐
Had difficulty going out for a meal?	☐	☐	☐	☐	☐	☐
Had difficulty using public transportation?	☐	☐	☐	☐	☐	☐
Felt not in control of your life?	☐	☐	☐	☐	☐	☐
Felt frustrated?	☐	☐	☐	☐	☐	☐

(continued)

TABLE 4.3 The Health-Related Quality of Life Questionnaire for Patients with PSP (PSP-QoL) (*continued*)

In the last 4 weeks, have you:	No problem	Slight problem	Moderate problem	Marked problem	Extreme problem	Not applicable
Felt a bit down, sad, or depressed?	☐	☐	☐	☐	☐	☐
Felt pessimistic about the future?	☐	☐	☐	☐	☐	☐
Felt anxious?	☐	☐	☐	☐	☐	☐
Felt isolated?	☐	☐	☐	☐	☐	☐
Had difficulty sleeping not due to problems moving?	☐	☐	☐	☐	☐	☐
Found yourself crying?	☐	☐	☐	☐	☐	☐
Become more withdrawn?	☐	☐	☐	☐	☐	☐
Felt stuck at home?	☐	☐	☐	☐	☐	☐
Felt embarrassed in public?	☐	☐	☐	☐	☐	☐
Felt you cannot show your feelings?	☐	☐	☐	☐	☐	☐
Found your personality is different from before your illness?	☐	☐	☐	☐	☐	☐
Felt the relationship with your spouse or partner has changed?	☐	☐	☐	☐	☐	☐
Seen family less than before you had this condition?	☐	☐	☐	☐	☐	☐
Had problems with your memory?	☐	☐	☐	☐	☐	☐
Found yourself repeating things a lot?	☐	☐	☐	☐	☐	☐
Found your thinking is slower than before the illness?	☐	☐	☐	☐	☐	☐
Found your thinking is muddled?	☐	☐	☐	☐	☐	☐
Felt confused?	☐	☐	☐	☐	☐	☐
Felt not motivated to do things?	☐	☐	☐	☐	☐	☐
Found it difficult to make decisions?	☐	☐	☐	☐	☐	☐

Please make sure you've checked one box for each question.

Experiencing any illness has an effect on one's life. Please indicate how satisfied you feel overall with your life at the moment by putting a cross on the line between 0 and 100.

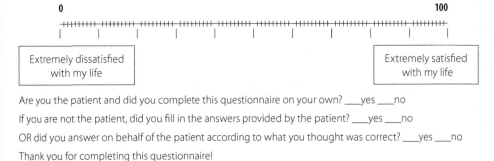

Are you the patient and did you complete this questionnaire on your own? ___yes ___no

If you are not the patient, did you fill in the answers provided by the patient? ___yes ___no

OR did you answer on behalf of the patient according to what you thought was correct? ___yes ___no

Thank you for completing this questionnaire!

about 15 minutes in most PSP patient/caregiver pairs, makes it difficult to include in a brief clinical follow-up encounter along with a physical exam measure such as the PSPRS or UPDRS motor section. However, the PSP-QoL is also designed to be completed at home by patient and caregiver, a major virtue. The scale appears as Table 4.3.

A REVIEW

In 2016, a critical review of 27 rating scales used in PSP was published by Hall et al (Disclaimer: I was a minor coauthor.) It concluded that the PSPRS, the motor portion of the UPDRS and the Frontal Assessment Battery, met criteria as "recommended" because they met all 3 of the protocol's criteria: (1) published use in PSP populations; (2) clinimetric properties that had been evaluated, found adequate, and published; and (3) published use by groups other than their original developers. Of those 3 scales, the PSPRS is the only one specific to PSP. Seven other scales received a "suggested" rating because they met 2 of the 3 criteria. They are the NNIPPS-PPS, PSP-QoL, Hoehn-Yahr stage, Dementia Rating Scale, Mini-Mental Status Examination, Neuropsychiatric Inventory, and the European Quality of Life Five-Dimensional Scale (EQ-5D). The NNIPPS-PPS Scale and the PSP-QoL were mentioned by Hall et al as having potential to be "recommended" but require more evaluation.

Clinical Spectrum 5

In 1963 and 1964, Drs. Steele, Richardson, and Olszewski described 7 patients with a nearly uniform set of clinical and pathological findings. The following few decades improved little on that clinicopathologic picture. Both the clinical syndrome and the anatomic pathology were hard to mistake for anything else. Researchers entertained notions of soon finding a discrete environmental cause of this sporadic, seemingly unvarying disorder.

But gradually, trouble arose. Autopsy-confirmed cases of progressive supranuclear palsy (PSP) without eye movement defects were published. A few familial cases appeared. A wide range of cognitive defects was described. Although the onset age variance of PSP is not nearly as wide as that of Parkinson disease, it was found to be wide enough to suggest underlying etiologic variability, with the youngest autopsy-proven case having suffered symptom onset at age 43 years. The cardinal clinical features' order of appearance and their relative severities were found to vary.

Starting as early as the 1970s, observant neurologists noticed that while most patients with PSP varied within a well-defined set of bounds easily recognizable by Drs. Steele et al, a minority took a very different path to the diagnosis. They were initially diagnosed as having Parkinson disease but with only modest levodopa response and little or no tremor. The puzzled neurologist may have suspected a diagnosis of vascular parkinsonism. The result of what we now call "small vessel ischemic disease" had been described by Critchley in 1929 in autopsies. However, it was difficult to diagnose in the living patient, as magnetic resonance imaging (MRI) was not yet available and computed tomography (CT) scanning in the 1970s had insufficient resolution. Another diagnostic possibility that our discouraged neurologist would have considered for such patients was normal-pressure hydrocephalus, which had been described at about the same time as PSP, in 1965 (Adams et al, 1965). However, that condition's enlarged ventricles without sulcal enlargement were easily ruled out by a CT scan, which became widely available a few years later.

Then, at a point 4 or 5 years into our unusual patient's symptomatic course, the syndrome so vividly described by Steele et al coalesced. Our puzzled neurologist now realized that the patient had evolved over 3 or 4 years into someone with a disinhibited manner, an overinnervated face, riveted eyes, growling dysarthria, upright posture, and neck rigidity out of proportion to limb bradykinesia. The neurologist realized that many of these features had been present before but perhaps not to this degree. Perhaps the neurologist had been asking himself, "How can I get this patient to respond better to levodopa?" rather than "What diagnosis other than Parkinson disease might this patient have?" (I confess that despite the benefit of having seen hundreds of patients with PSP over 4 decades, I occasionally cling to my diagnosis of "levodopa-resistant Parkinson disease" too long.)

In 1998, I wrote a book chapter on PSP that included the following description of what would later be called "PSP-parkinsonism" (Golbe, 1998). It is important to mention that I neither originated this observation nor had adequate autopsy support for it.

> One classic presentation of PSP occurs in the patient with what appears to be nontremorous PD. The patient may even respond modestly to levodopa for a year or two. At about the time the clinician realizes that the levodopa response is less than expected in PD, he detects more postural instability, dysarthria and dysphagia than PD produces for the duration of illness. Often, the clinician suspects PSP but fails to detect restriction of vertical eye movement and continues to call the illness PD. At this stage, the vertical supranuclear palsy is often very subtle or absent.

In 2005, that observation received systematic and autopsy-confirmed support, and the notion of a unitary PSP officially died. In that year, in what is probably the most important paper on PSP since Steele et al, Williams and colleagues (2005) described 2 clinical PSP phenotypes among their 105 cases of autopsy-confirmed PSP. They called them "Richardson syndrome" (RS) and "PSP-parkinsonism" (PSP-P). The 54% with RS had the syndrome described by Steele et al, with an emphasis on falls, vertical gaze palsy, frontal dementia, and abnormal saccadic physiology. The 32% with PSP-P emphasized bradykinesia, asymmetric onset, tremor, dystonia, and, initially, levodopa responsiveness. The remaining 14% were not classifiable. Importantly, these clusters of features were just that—groups of items that occurred together in the same patients. This suggests that while they may both be PSP by its current autopsy-based definition, they are actually 2 different diseases at some level.

Variation in PSP was also discovered at the molecular level. The gene encoding tau protein (the MAPT gene) has 2 major variants in humans called the H1 and H2 haplotypes. In European-derived populations, about 60% of individuals are homozygous for H1, 34% are H1/H2 heterozygous, and 7% are homozygous for H2. But in the population with autopsy-confirmed PSP, it is 88% H1/H1, 12% H1/H2, and none (or a rare case) H2/H2. Yet this relationship, as shown by Williams et al, is true only for Richardson syndrome! It is just that in their series, PSP-RS accounts for more than 50% of all PSP, so its statistical influence holds up even when all PSP is considered.

Another observation of Williams et al suggests a second difference between PSP-RS and PSP-P at the molecular level. It concerns the ratio of 4-repeat to 3-repeat tau. First, some background for the nonspecialist: normal tau protein binds to the cell's microtubules, promoting their maintenance and growth. Each tau molecule has either 3 or 4 "microtubule binding domains," where it can attach itself. In normal adult human brain, the ratio of "4-repeat" to "3-repeat" tau is about 1:1. But in PSP, it is about 3:1. In the cases of Williams et al, the ratio was 2.84:1 for PSP-RS and 1.63:1 for PSP-P, a statistically significant difference ($P = .002$).

So there is a second PSP that satisfies the pathologic criteria for PSP but looks a lot like Parkinson disease and does not share the strong tendency of most PSP for its most important known genetic association or for an important feature of its aggregating protein.

Early evidence shows that PSP-RS and PSP-P differ in the anatomical structures bearing the brunt of the damage, as one would predict given their differences in clinical deficits. Another demonstration of the wide pathologic variation of PSP is the 2008 report of "incidental PSP" described in the chapter on epidemiology. The question, then, is whether PSP could be more than one molecular process. If so, does each PSP-causing molecular process have its own ultimate etiology? And if that is the case, will each have its own specific prevention, treatment, or cure?

PSP-PARKINSONISM VS PSP-RICHARDSON SYNDROME

Factor analysis in the seminal 2005 report by Williams et al showed that cognitive loss, postural instability, falls, supranuclear gaze palsy, and abnormal saccadic or pursuit movements tended to cluster in the RS group, while asymmetry, bradykinesia, tremor, dystonia, and levodopa responsiveness clustered among the PSP-P group. Rigidity, pyramidal findings, dysphagia, visual disturbances, dyskinesia, and dysarthria were frequent in both groups without a statistically significant predilection for either.

Through the end of 2017, a total of 10 presentations, or phenotypes, of pathologically proven PSP have been published. In general, the picture begins in its atypical way and evolves over a period of years to include the more typical features of Richardson syndrome. The prevalence of the various presentations is difficult to measure because most of the published series include only a few patients without reference to a population denominator. Furthermore, because atypical cases are more likely to come to autopsy, it is difficult to estimate the population prevalence of atypical cases of PSP from autopsy series. Nevertheless, the "minority phenotypes" are described here in approximate descending order of prevalence.

PSP–PROGRESSIVE GAIT FREEZING

After PSP-P, the most common minority phenotype is PSP–progressive gait freezing (PSP-PGF), accounting for about 5% of PSP (Williams et al, 2007). In fact, most patients exhibiting only progressive gait freezing will eventually prove to have PSP and gait freezing has good predictive value for a diagnosis of PSP (Osaki et al, 2017). The central feature of PSP-PGF is loss of ability to continue ongoing gait, especially after a pause, during a turn or at a doorway threshold. In advanced cases, the patient cannot initiate gait at all. The picture also includes rapid micrographia and rapid, hypophonic speech as frequent or severe features. The anatomic location of the pathology in such cases differs from that of PSP-RS in showing less involvement of the pontine base and dentate nuclei of the cerebellum.

PSP–CORTICOBASAL SYNDROME

The next most common is probably PSP–corticobasal syndrome (PSP-CBS) (Ling et al, 2014). CBS as a clinical syndrome comprises highly asymmetric rigidity, bradykinesia, and apraxia, often with equally asymmetric dystonia, pyramidal findings, myoclonus, and cortical sensory signs such as astereognosis and agraphesthesia. Dysarthria can be prominent. Gaze palsy, postural instability, and cognitive loss tend to be later and milder than in PSP-RS. Aphasia and other focal abnormalities may also occur. Its most common pathologic underpinning is corticobasal degeneration, accounting for about half of all clinical cases of CBS. PSP pathology accounts for about 5% to 10% of the total. In PSP-CBS, the pathology shifts its emphasis to the cerebral cortex from the basal ganglia and brainstem loci of PSP-RS.

It is important to understand that just as the cellular pathology of PSP can produce multiple clinical phenotypes depending on its anatomic distribution, the pathology called corticobasal degeneration (CBD) has its own clinical spectrum. Only about a third of patients with CBD at autopsy had clinical CBS during life. Perhaps 5% to 10% had Richardson syndrome. It is also relevant that pathologies of CBD and PSP-RS are both among the dozens of disorders based on aggregation of 4-repeat tau. (Normal adult human tau has equal proportions of 3- and 4-repeat types.) There may also be at least 1 genetic risk factor in common, a variant in or near the MOBP gene, which encodes a component of myelin. But the uniquely identifying form of tauopathy in PSP is tufted astrocytes, while in CBD, it is astrocytic plaques, ballooned neurons, and achromatic neurons. Nevertheless, cases of CBD often include PSP copathology. Clearly, the relationship of PSP and CBD as both clinical and pathologic entities is complex and only partly understood.

PSP-BEHAVIORAL-VARIANT FRONTOTEMPORAL DEMENTIA

PSP-behavioral-variant frontotemporal dementia (PSP-bvFTD) features disinhibition, irritability, apathy, and loss of empathy for others, along with impairment in frontal "executive" functions such as ability to maintain attention, to follow instructions, to shift tasks on command, and to inhibit an ongoing action when appropriate (Donker Kaat et al, 2007). This is the core of the cognitive and behavioral deficits in Richardson syndrome, but when it appears first and remains worst, the term *PSP-bvFTD* is appropriate.

PSP NONFLUENT/AGRAMMATIC VARIANT OF PRIMARY PROGRESSIVE APHASIA

PSP–nonfluent/agrammatic variant of primary progressive aphasia (PSP-nfaPPA) is another rare presentation of PSP pathology (Santos-Santos et al, 2016). Here, speech is halting, with poor grammar, syntax, and phoneme pronunciation, but with normal comprehension and naming. A mirror-image variant, equally rare, called semantic-variant primary progressive aphasia (svPPA), features difficulty in naming with reduced vocabulary but with normal grammar and syntax. Together, PSP-svPPA and PSP-nfaPPA are sometimes referred to in the literature as PSP–speech/language disorder (PSP-SL).

PSP-CEREBELLAR

Cerebellar involvement in PSP (PSP-C) has been known since the original pathologic description of "grumose degeneration" (a form of tauopathy) of the cerebellar dentate by Olszewski, Steele and Richardson in 1963. The classic lurching gait of Richardson syndrome has a cerebellar appearance, the dysarthria has an ataxic component in many cases, and the ocular square-wave jerks of PSP occur commonly in cerebellar disease. Nevertheless, important cerebellar involvement was an exclusionary criterion in all of the proposed sets of PSP clinical criteria through the publication of the now-standard National Institute of Neurological Disorders and Stroke and Society for Progressive Supranuclear Palsy (NINDS-SPSP) criteria in 1996. The purpose was to exclude patients with multiple-system atrophy and some of the spinocerebellar ataxias, which may otherwise mimic PSP clinically. But in 2009, Kanazawa et al described PSP where involvement of the cerebellum exceeded that of the midbrain and where the truncal and limb ataxia was an early and prominent feature (Kanazawa 2013). Three of their 22 autopsied cases with PSP had this variant. Since then, PSP-C has been seen outside of Japan, albeit at a lower prevalence. At the Mayo Clinic, Koga et al in 2016 found PSP-C in just 1 of their 100 consecutive autopsied cases with good clinical data (Koga et al, 2016).

For a clinician, it is difficult to distinguish PSP-C from the cerebellar form of multiple-system atrophy (MSA-C). The onset age of PSP-C is later than that of MSA, consistent with the generally later onset of PSP than of MSA. PSP-C displays more falling and more supranuclear gaze deficits. MSA-C displays dysautonomia in the first 2 years of illness in 90% of cases, while the same was true for none of the 3 cases of PSP-C in the series of Kanazawa et al (2009), where that clinical information was available.

PSP–PRIMARY LATERAL SCLEROSIS

The pathology of PSP can also produce the clinical picture of primary lateral sclerosis. Josephs et al (2006) found that in 9 of 289 autopsied cases of PSP (3%), typical PSP pathology heavily involved the motor cortex. The clinical picture of PSP–primary lateral sclerosis (PSP-PLS) was highly asymmetric and resembled that of CBS but with little or no cortical sensory loss, dystonia, or myoclonus.

PSP–OCULAR MOTOR AND PSP–POSTURAL INSTABILITY

Perhaps unsurprisingly given the cardinal features of PSP-RS, PSP can also take the form of a relatively pure ocular motor syndrome or a syndrome of severe postural instability (Respondek et al, 2014). However, reported cases are very sparse to date. These have been designated PSP–ocular motor and PSP–postural instability.

EPIDEMIOLOGY OF THE PHENOTYPES

Armed with these new insights, Respondek et al in 2014 reviewed clinical records of 100 cases of autopsy-proven PSP. PSP–Richardson syndrome accounted for only 24%, PSP–parkinsonism for 19%, PSP–postural instability for 18%, PSP–frontotemporal dementia for 12%, PSP–ocular motor for 7%, and PSP–corticobasal syndrome for 7%. They were unable to classify 13%. The contrast of PSP-RS as 24% of their series with the 54% of the 2005 series of Williams et al may demonstrate the progress in understanding the spectrum of PSP over that decade or may simply demonstrate a difference in diagnostic criteria or in brain bank referral bias. Other large autopsy-based series with excellent clinical records are needed to resolve this disparity.

Although there is a statistically valid clustering of clinical symptoms in PSP-RS relative to PSP-P, a result since confirmed by others, the same cannot be said for the other PSP phenotypes with respect to one another or to PSP-RS or PSP-P. The question therefore arises: are these variants different "diseases" at some fundamental pathogenetic or etiologic level? Williams et al did find PSP-RS far more likely than PSP-P to feature 4-repeat tau predominance, the MAPT H1 haplotype, and male gender, as described above. However, these findings have not been replicated, and no other such biomarker differences have been reported for the other PSP phenotypes. The available autopsy studies have shown the same pathology for all of the phenotypes in differing anatomic locations. Of potential help here are imaging data, where 1 small study to date shows differences among some of the PSP variants. However, those few cases and the other available biomarker data on the PSP variants remain insufficient to conclude whether the conditions are statistically separable or merely different points in a smoothly varying spectrum. The possibility therefore remains that all (or most) of the clinical phenotypes are merely blinkered views of pieces of the same diverse disease. The newer genetic and epigenetic technology may clarify that situation very soon.

Until the pathogenetic commonalities among the various PSP phenotypes are better understood, neuroprotection trials—those aimed at targets fundamental to the pathogenesis of cell loss rather than merely at ameliorating the symptoms—will continue to recruit only patients with Richardson syndrome. The justification is that the pathogenesis of other phenotypes may not include the same drug target, at least not as a rate-limiting step.

Differential Diagnosis 6

MICROSCOPICAL FEATURES

As promised in the preface, this book will not discuss details of the neuropathology of progressive supranuclear palsy (PSP). But a chapter on differential diagnosis should start by pointing out that definite PSP can only be diagnosed at autopsy. On gross inspection, the neuropathologist finds atrophy of the subthalamic nuclei, globus pallidus (particularly the interna), substantia nigra, pontine and midbrain tegmentum, pretectal area, and periaqueductal gray (Hauw et al, 1994). At the cellular level, PSP is distinguished from its mimics by the absence of not only amyloid plaques but also neuritic plaques that occur in other tauopathies. Tau aggregation occurs in the form of neurofibrillary tangles in neurons, neuropil threads in dendrites, coiled bodies in oligodendrocytes, and "tufts" in astrocytes. There is also tau-positive "grumose degeneration" in the dentate of the cerebellum (Dickson, 1999). Immunostaining reveals that the aggregated tau in all of these locations is hyperphosphorylated.

The tables show the clinical differential diagnosis of PSP from 4 different perspectives. Table 6.1 shows causes of vertical gaze palsy, with or without other features of PSP. Table 6.2 shows the major neurodegenerative parkinsonian disorders that are the frequent diagnostic considerations in everyday practice. Table 6.3 puts PSP in the context of the other major tauopathies. The text describes the most important or treatable differential diagnostic considerations in more detail.

TABLE 6.1 Adult-onset diseases that may produce vertical (up or down) supranuclear gaze palsy

Disease class	
Degenerative	PSP
	Multiple-system atrophy
	Dementia with Lewy bodies
	Frontotemporal dementia with ubiquitin staining
	Frontotemporal dementia with tau staining
	PD (only upgaze affected)
	Pallidal degeneration
	Lytico-bodig
	Huntington disease
	Creutzfeldt-Jakob disease
	Amyotrophic lateral sclerosis
	Motor neuron disease with congophilic angiopathy
Vascular	Lacunar states ("vascular PSP")
	Cerebral autosomal dominant arteriopathy with subcortical infarcts and leukoencephalopathy (CADASIL)
	Postaortic surgery
Structural	Third ventricular enlargement
	Pineal region masses
Metabolic/storage	Niemann-Pick disease type C
	Wilson disease
	B12 deficiency
	Wernicke encephalopathy
	Adult-onset Tay-Sachs disease (hypometric saccades)
Infectious	Whipple disease
	Neurosyphilis
Immune	Antiphospholipid syndrome
	Paraneoplastic syndromes
Toxic	Guadeloupean tauopathy

TABLE 6.2 The major degenerative parkinsonisms

	PSP	Parkinson disease	Corticobasal degeneration	Multiple-system atrophy	Dementia with Lewy bodies	Behavioral variant frontotemporal dementia
Marquee feature	Brainstem	Rest tremor	Asymmetry, apraxia	Dysautonomia, ataxia	Hallucinations, early dementia, or mood change	Disinhibition
Motor first/worst	++	++	++	++	−	−
Dementia first/worst	+	−	−	−	++	+++
Major autonomic features	−	+	−	+++	++	−
Good motor levodopa response	+	+++	−	+	++	−
Prevalence per 100,000 population	5–6	150	<1	4	Approx. 100	20

Note: Absent − ; Mild + ; Moderate ++ ; Marked +++

PARKINSON DISEASE

To the practiced eye, PSP–Richardson syndrome (PSP-RS) differs dramatically from Parkinson disease (PD). In PD, the posture is stooped and the stride is regular, with a normal, narrow base, and is performed with an abundance of caution. The posture in PSP is stooped in only a minority, erect in the majority and hyper-erect in 10%. The stride is irregular, with a base that is wide at times and scissoring at others, and plunges ahead seemingly oblivious to the risk.

In PD, the limbs and neck are approximately equally rigid, and a tapping task loses amplitude over the first 10 or 15 cycles. In PSP, the neck is more rigid than the limbs in most cases, and the tapping task starts with a low amplitude that does not lessen over the duration of the task. The speech of PD, discussed in the chapter on dysarthria, is soft and fast, while in PSP, it is often explosive, slow, and irregular.

TABLE 6.3 Tauopathies

Alzheimer disease	Neurodegeneration with brain iron accumulation
Amyotrophic-parkinsonism-dementia complex of Guam (lytico-bodig)	Niemann-Pick disease type C
Argyrophilic grain disease	Non-Guamanian motor neuron disease with neurofibrillary tangles
Chronic traumatic encephalopathy	
Diffuse neurofibrillary tangles with calcification	Pick disease
Down syndrome	Postencephalitic parkinsonism
Familial British dementia	Prion protein cerebral amyloid angiopathy
Familial Danish dementia	Progressive subcortical gliosis
Frontotemporal dementia and parkinsonism linked to chromosome 17 mutations (FTDP-17)	PSP
Frontotemporal lobal degeneration (some cases)	SLC9A6-related mental retardation
	Subacute sclerosing panencephalopathy
Gerstmann-Sträussler-Scheinker disease	Tangle-only dementia
Guadeloupean tauopathy	White matter tauopathy with globular glial inclusions
Myotonic dystrophy	

Tremor in PD is predominantly at rest and is complex, involving multiple joints oscillating in multiple planes, the classic pill-rolling being one example. In PSP, the tremor occurs with posture and/or action and is simple in its anatomy and geometry. It occurs in about 25% of cases, mostly those with the PSP-parkinsonism phenotype.

In PD, range of gaze is normal, particularly horizontally, but in PSP, there is no unnecessary eye movement, and when attention must be directed horizontally, the head is rotated before, or instead of, the eyes.

The clinical course is faster in PSP than in PD, even correcting for its lesser levodopa response. The order of acquisition of deficits in PD typically starts with tremor or a hemi-bradykinesia, while in PSP, the first problem is almost always postural instability or behavioral change, occasionally a brainstem issue.

The cognitive loss of PD is typically absent for the first few years and, when it does occur, is diffuse, involving parietal, temporal, and frontal areas. In PSP, the affection is mostly frontal, sooner in the course and includes levels of both apathy and disinhibition rarely seen in PD.

Other differences between PD and PSP are described in their respective chapters. The PSP-parkinsonism (PSP-P) phenotype more closely conforms to the picture in PD early in its course and only later converges with PSP-RS.

MULTIPLE-SYSTEM ATROPHY

Multiple-system atrophy (MSA) is slightly less common than PSP, and its average onset age is 54 years, a decade younger. Median survival is similar to that of PSP at approximately 7 years. MSA features some combination of rigidity/ bradykinesia, dysautonomia, and cerebellar features. There may also be gaze palsies, dysphagia, sleep disturbance, ventilatory arrhythmia, bizarre dystonia, and moderate frontal dementia.

MSA can include vertical gaze palsy, but unlike in PSP, horizontal eye movement problems such as slow saccades, gaze limitation, and nystagmus are far more important in MSA than the vertical component. Square-wave jerks, which are horizontal intrusions during ocular fixation that arise from the disruption of cerebellar circuits, are nearly universal in PSP, but occur in about two-thirds of patients with MSA (Anderson and MacAskill, 2013). Rapidly progressive parkinsonism with severe postural instability and poor levodopa response can give the misimpression of PSP if the other features of MSA are not carefully sought. Magnetic resonance imaging (MRI) findings of cerebellar and pontine atrophy along with pontine gliosis in a "hot cross bun sign" pattern can distinguish MSA from PSP in the middle and later stages (see Figures 16.8b and 16.8c). This MRI sign is not specific for MSA, occurring as well in some of the hereditary spinocerebellar ataxias (SCAs), particularly SCAs 1, 2, and 3.

As a historical note, the predominantly cerebellar form of MSA (MSA-C) was once termed *sporadic olivopontocerebellar atrophy*, and the parkinsonian form (MSA-P) was called *striato-nigral degeneration*. MSA of either type with dysautonomia was called *Shy-Drager syndrome*. In 1989, the 3 conditions were found to share a newly identified protein aggregate dubbed *glial cytoplasmic inclusions* (GCI). The 3 MSA types differ in their anatomic distribution of GCIs and cell loss but with continuous variation among the types that corresponds to their combinations of clinical deficits. In 1998, a few months after the discovery that the Lewy bodies of Parkinson disease comprised mostly alpha-synuclein, the same was first reported for the inclusions of MSA. However, the latter are structurally different from Lewy bodies and occur in glia rather than neurons.

As can be inferred from the above, the term *Shy-Drager syndrome* is now obsolete. It should be avoided completely, as it is merely an ill-defined region on the MSA clinical spectrum. One still sees the term erroneously used in medical records (although not in the published literature) to refer to any combination of autonomic dysfunction with motor parkinsonism, including Parkinson disease.

DEMENTIA WITH LEWY BODIES

PSP and dementia with Lewy bodies (DLB) both affect the brain in widespread anatomic fashion, with the dopaminergic substantia nigra an important center of pathology and vertical gaze often involved. Both disorders cause dementia, although that of DLB is a diffuse dementia with an important amnestic and/or affective component, while that of PSP is predominantly frontal and features apathy. Distinguishing DLB best from PSP is psychosis independent of dopaminergic drugs. Other helpful distinguishing features of DLB are its useful, sustained response to levodopa, its autonomic involvement and its fluctuations in consciousness lasting minutes to hours.

MULTI-INFARCT STATES AND
NORMAL-PRESSURE HYDROCEPHALUS

The most important single reason to obtain a brain MRI in patients with suspected PSP is to rule out a vascular state or normal-pressure hydrocephalus.

Multiple lacunar infarctions in various combinations of locations can mimic many neurodegenerative conditions, including PSP in rare cases. By clinical exam, "vascular PSP" may be indistinguishable from PSP but by MRI shows high T2 signal involving the basal ganglia and upper brainstem. The cross-sectional areas of the midbrain and superior cerebellar peduncle are more atrophic in PSP than in its vascular mimics. The dopamine transporter (DaT) scan is typically normal in vascular states but abnormal in PSP although in the United States, the paucity of supporting literature has prompted regulators and payors to not recognize this differential diagnosis as justification for the scan.

In normal-pressure hydrocephalus (NPH) the gait apraxia, "subcortical" dementia, and urinary incontinence may mimic those features of PSP. The classic picture of NPH starts with "magnetic gait" typically but not always comprising external rotation at the hips and poor floor clearance. The next sign is urinary urgency and incontinence and, finally, dementia. Falls, supranuclear gaze, and brainstem deficits do not occur more than expected for age. If dementia appears first, one must strongly suspect a degenerative cause, with PSP leading the list. Two series describe patients transiently responding to shunting who later developed diagnosable signs of PSP (Morariu, 1979; Curran and Lang, 1994), and I have seen several such cases myself.

The concept of both vascular parkinsonism and NPH have recently been called into question on grounds of poor clinicopathological support (Espay et al, 2017; Vizcarra et al, 2015). Neurodegenerative disorders, including PSP, may explain many cases of vascular parkinsonism and NPH. For these reasons I encourage our institution's neurosurgeons to allow me or another movement disorders neurologist to evaluate patients referred to them with a diagnosis of NPH even before they schedule a diagnostic lumbar drainage procedure.

CORTICOBASAL DEGENERATION

Corticobasal degeneration (CBD) is a pathologically defined condition very similar to PSP at the cellular and molecular levels. Its classic clinical presentation, occurring in about 40% of cases, is corticobasal syndrome (CBS), which features highly asymmetric motor features of limb apraxia, bradykinesia, dystonia, rigidity, myoclonus, and pyramidal signs. CBS also frequently includes cortical sensory loss in the form of agraphesthesia, tested by asking the patient to identify numbers traced on the palm with eyes closed, and astereognosis, tested by identifying common objects placed in the hand. The asymmetry of these deficits is the most important single point differentiating PSP from CBD (Boeve et al, 2003).

About 5% of pathologic CBD presents with Richardson syndrome (CBD-RS), the classic clinical phenotype of PSP. Distinguishing CBD-RS from PSP-RS may be difficult, relying principally on motor asymmetry as a clue to CBD as the underlying pathology. Apraxia and limb dystonia are nearly universal in CBD but occur in about half of patients with PSP. However, when either does occur in PSP, it is almost always highly asymmetric. The apraxia of CBD is more likely than that of PSP to be severe, distal and intransitive (that is, involving non-tool-using actions such as saluting rather than tool-using actions such as hammering) (Zadikoff et al, 2005).

After CBD, the next most common pathology underlying CBS is PSP, followed by Alzheimer disease and dementia with Lewy bodies. Rare patients with very rapidly progressive CBS may prove to have a prion disease such as Creutzfeldt-Jacob disease (CJD), variant CJD, or fatal familial insomnia. Others may have Wernicke encephalopathy or a paraneoplastic condition such as anti-voltage-gated potassium channel encephalopathy.

WHIPPLE DISEASE

This chronic bacterial infection may rarely involve any of multiple brain areas but is primary to the small intestine with malabsorption but also causes arthritis, pericarditis, uveitis, and vasculitis. Onset age ranges from early childhood through the 50s, with a peak in the 30s and 40s with a marked male predominance. Neurological features in a small proportion of cases include severe vertical gaze palsy and, in a few reported cases, bradykinesia. However, the other central nervous system (CNS) features of Whipple disease are not particularly suggestive of PSP. They feature facial movements termed *oculomasticatory myorhythmia*, amnestic dementia, hemiparesis with pyramidal signs, marked ataxia, and meningeal signs (Compain et al, 2013). On MRI, Whipple disease usually shows contrast ring–enhancing nodules or larger masses resembling tumors or abscesses.

The National Institute of Neurological Disorders and Stroke and Society for Progressive Supranuclear Palsy (NINDS-SPSP) criteria for the clinical diagnosis of PSP list Whipple disease among the diagnostic alternatives that must be ruled out "when indicated." The screening test polymerase chain reaction for *Tropheryma whipplei* DNA uses blood or cerebrospinal fluid (CSF). However, the disease is extremely rare, and neurological involvement is even more so. My informal survey of senior leaders of clinical PSP referral centers revealed no cases of Whipple disease found among their collective experience of hundreds of patients presenting with signs suggesting PSP. The new revision of PSP diagnostic criteria continues this recommendation, now providing examples of "suggestive features" that would prompt ordering the test, including the non–CNS features mentioned above.

NIEMANN-PICK DISEASE TYPE C

The diagnostic criteria for PSP require the neurological symptoms to have started by age 40 years. There has never been a published, autopsy-proven case of PSP with onset before that age, but the reason to impose the age minimum is to rule out Niemann-Pick disease type C (NPC). This lysosomal storage disease results from deficiency of acid sphingomyelinase and occurs in 1 of 120,000 live births. It typically manifests during infancy or childhood with vertical gaze palsy and splenomegaly followed by general developmental failure and death by the 20s. Adult onset is rare, occurring in the 20s through early 50s. As in infants, vertical gaze palsy is the most common neurological manifestation, but frontal dementia, psychosis, seizures, myoclonus, ataxia, and dystonia may also occur, occasionally without gaze palsy (Salsano et al, 2012). Splenomegaly is nearly universal, and hepatomegaly with abnormal liver function occurs in the majority. Confirmatory diagnosis is via skin biopsy with staining of cultured skin fibroblasts with filipin, which specifically stains cholesterol. Sequencing of the NPC1 gene shows a mutation in 95% of cases and in the NPC2 gene in 5%. This test is commercially available and can further confirm the diagnosis and assist in genetic counseling for the family.

It is important not to miss a diagnosis of NPC because treatment with miglustat may be available. It acts by inhibiting the synthesis of glucosphingolipids, slowing or stabilizing disease progression. At present, the drug is approved in the United States only for Gaucher disease and in several other countries for NPC.

FRONTOTEMPORAL LOBAR DEGENERATION WITH MOTOR NEURON DISEASE

Several times a year, my departmental colleagues in neuromuscular disease refer a patient to me who was referred to them as having possible amyotrophic lateral sclerosis. That suspicion was typically based on the gait change and dysarthria. But none of the diagnostic signs of motor neuron disease were in fact present, and the patient in fact fulfilled criteria for PSP or, more commonly, corticobasal degeneration.

The opposite error can also occur, where a patient referred to a movement center as having PSP because of frontal dementia and gait problems in fact has the rare condition of frontotemporal lobar degeneration with motor neuron disease (FTLD-MND). Diagnostic tipoffs would be marked hyper-reflexia, focal weakness, and signs of denervation on electromyography. To make matters more complicated, a PSP phenotype and a corticobasal syndrome phenotype can occur in FTLD (Hoglinger et al, 2017). When a patient with either of those syndromes also has severe language disturbance, severe dysexecutive dementia, or changes in personality early in the course, the diagnosis may be FTLD-PSP or FTLD-CBS.

OTHER TREATABLE, NONDEGENERATIVE CONDITIONS

Some conditions can cause the appearance of parkinsonism, with slowed or sparse movement and rigidity and absence of a levodopa benefit, prompting suspicion of PSP.

The psychomotor slowing of depression and the rigidity of catatonia fall under this rubric. An important part of the interview of anyone with parkinsonism should include inquiry into diagnosed or undiagnosed psychiatric symptoms. Another important goal of such inquiry, of course, is to exclude neuroleptic parkinsonism, which can be treated by reducing the neuroleptic dosage or by replacing it with quetiapine or clozapine, neuroleptics with little parkinsonogenic potential. Hypothyroidism can produce generalized slowing and paucity of motor activity. A dystonic tremor can also mimic parkinsonism, with limited mobility of the dystonic segments. An important clue is that the tremor of parkinsonism is pendular, with both the "to" and the "fro" phases of equal velocity, while a dystonic tremor has faster and slower phases. A final example is a frozen shoulder, where muscle spasm and pain may mimic the asymmetric onset of parkinsonism. However, the more typical confusion is in the opposite direction, where degenerative parkinsonism presenting asymmetrically is diagnosed and operated upon as an orthopedic issue.

All of these examples above are highly treatable and the clinician is well advised not to accept an existing diagnosis of PSP at face value.

Diagnostic Criteria 7

THE NINDS-SPSP CRITERIA

In 1996, Dr. Irene Litvan organized an international collaboration of neuropathologists to contribute a total of 24 cases with autopsy-confirmed progressive supranuclear palsy (PSP) and 59 with diagnoses on the differential diagnosis of PSP. All 83 had excellent clinical records available. The non-PSP cases comprised 15 with multiple-system atrophy, 14 with Lewy body dementia, 11 with Parkinson disease, 11 with corticobasal degeneration, and 8 with Pick disease (now considered one type of frontotemporal lobar degeneration). The same project organized a panel of experienced clinicians (disclaimer: including myself) to use the recorded clinical data to create 2 sets of clinical criteria.

The clinical and pathological PSP criteria sets are called the NINDS-SPSP Criteria because the National Institute of Neurological Disorders and Stroke together with the Society for PSP (since renamed CurePSP) sponsored the project. However, they have been informally and deservedly dubbed the "Litvan criteria" and remain the worldwide standard for research and clinical care in PSP.

One result of the National Institute of Neurological Disorders and Stroke and Society for Progressive Supranuclear Palsy (NINDS-SPSP) project was the delineation of pathologic criteria for PSP, called "definite" PSP. The 2 levels of clinically applicable criteria received the terms *probable* and *possible* PSP. The first maximizes specificity for use in clinical trials or in evaluations of diagnostic markers or causal factors, where exclusion of non-PSP is paramount. The "possible" criteria, on the other hand, are designed for sensitivity in epidemiological or medical economic studies, where full case ascertainment in a population would be desirable, even at the cost of including a few false positives.

The "probable" criteria's specificity proved to be 100% and the sensitivity only 50%. The "possible" criteria's sensitivity was a very useful 83% but at the cost of reducing the specificity to 93%. A subsequent study using 47 autopsy-proven cases from the UK Parkinson's Brain Bank found a positive predictive value (PPV) of 100% for both probable and possible criteria applied at the first clinic visit. These fell only to 84% and 83% by the last clinic visit. This favorable outcome must, however, be viewed in light of the same assessment for 4 previously published sets of PSP criteria, which all had 100% PPV at the first visit and ranged from 78% to 91% by the last visit (Osaki et al, 2004; Osaki et al 2002).

The interrater agreement for the NINDS-SPSP criteria has a kappa score of 0.82, where 0.61 to 0.80 is "substantial," 0.81 to 0.99 is "almost perfect," and 1.0 is perfect. This is testament to their simplicity and ease of use (Lopez et al, 1999).

The NINDS-SPSP criteria appear in Table 7.1. Both possible and probable criteria require symptom onset at age 40 years or later, a progressive course, and absence of specific evidence of other diagnostic possibilities. The "possible" criteria allow either vertical gaze palsy or a combination of slow vertical saccades with falls in the first year of symptoms. The "probable" criteria require both vertical gaze palsy and falls in the first year (later revised to 2 years). *Gaze palsy* is defined in these criteria as less than 50% of the normal saccadic amplitude and *falls* as including events where a helper or object in the room prevents the patient from making contact with the floor.

The criteria publication helpfully offers several "supportive criteria" to assist the clinician but does not impose them as requirements. They include symmetric akinesia that is predominantly proximal; abnormal neck posture, especially retrocollis; poor or absent levodopa response; early dysphagia and dysarthria; and early cognitive difficulties such as apathy, abstraction difficulty, verbal influency, utilization/imitation behavior, and frontal release signs.

The NINDS-SPSP criteria also specify 8 mandatory exclusionary items. These are applicable to both the probable and possible criteria. Listed in Table 7.1, they reduce the likelihood of a false-positive diagnosis of PSP in cases of postencephalitic parkinsonism, corticobasal degeneration, dementia with Lewy bodies, Alzheimer disease, multiple-system atrophy, Parkinson disease (PD), Whipple disease, and structural abnormalities such as hydrocephalus, leukoencephalopathy, infarctions, tumors, or the isolated lobar atrophy seen on imaging in some cases of frontotemporal dementia.

TABLE 7.1 NINDS-SPSP criteria for the diagnosis of PSP

Possible PSP	Probable PSP
All 3 of these:	All 5 of these:
1. Gradually progressive disorder	1. Gradually progressive disorder
2. Onset at age 40 years or later	2. Onset at age 40 years or later
3. No evidence for competing diagnostic possibilities	3. No evidence for competing diagnostic possibilities
Plus either of these:	
4. Vertical gaze palsy	4. Vertical gaze palsy
or	5. Slowing of vertical saccades *and* prominent postural instability with falls in the first year
5. Slowing of vertical saccades *and* prominent postural instability with falls in the first year	

Criteria that would exclude PSP from consideration

1. Recent encephalitis

2. Alien limb syndrome, cortical sensory defects, or temporoparietal atrophy

3. Psychosis unrelated to dopaminergic treatment

4. Important cerebellar signs

5. Important unexplained dysautonomia

6. Severe, asymmetric parkinsonian signs

7. Relevant structural abnormality of basal ganglia on neuroimaging

8. Whipple disease on cerebrospinal fluid polymerase chain reaction, if indicated

Source: Litvan et al, 1996.

More recently, the criteria of Litvan et al (1996) were evaluated by Respondek et al (2013) using an autopsy-confirmed series of 98 cases with PSP and a "control" series of 18 with PD, 15 with corticobasal degeneration (CBD), and 13 with the parkinsonian form of multiple-system atrophy (MSA). The 3 latter disorders may reproduce the usual clinical differential diagnosis of PSP more faithfully than those used as controls by Litvan et al. The surprising result was that the "possible" criteria yielded a sensitivity of less than 20% during the first 3 years, rising to only 40% by the time of death. Other studies have found the figure to be as low as 14%. However, the specificity of the "probable" criteria was confirmed to be high, at over 90% for the entire disease course. The likely reason for the low sensitivity is that since the publication of the NINDS-SPSP criteria in 1996, multiple "minority phenotypes" of PSP have been described. They produce the same pathologic picture as the classic phenotype, which is now known as Richardson syndrome, but their clinical picture, especially in the first few years, can be very different.

THE MDS-PSP RESEARCH GROUP CRITERIA

Subsequently, the same group, led by Dr. Gunter Höglinger, initiated a project to update the NINDS-SPSP criteria to recognize the multiple newly described clinical PSP phenotypes and to recognize PSP–Richardson syndrome (PSP-RS) at an earlier stage of illness (Höglinger et al, 2017). It analyzed 462 papers using either autopsy confirmation or the NINDS-SPSP criteria and added 206 autopsy-confirmed cases of PSP, 54 with CBD, 51 with the parkinsonian form of MSA (MSA-P), 53 with PD, and 73 with behavioral-variant frontotemporal dementia (FTD). The project was supported by the Movement Disorder Society, and the result, called the MDS criteria for PSP, was published in 2017, and it appears in Tables 7.2 through 7.6.

These newest criteria define 3 levels of severity for each of 4 core clinical features: ocular motor dysfunction, postural instability, akinesia, and cognitive dysfunction. Details of each of these 12 definitions appear in Table 7.2. The criteria then list, in Table 7.3, combinations of the 12 necessary to apply 3 levels of clinical diagnostic certainty: "probable PSP," "possible PSP," and "suggestive of PSP." The last of these is an innovation intended for early identification of persons at risk for PSP who may be candidates for studies of primary prevention or early biomarkers.

The criteria start by requiring 3 "basic" criteria, shown in Table 7.4. The first is that the disorder cannot have a clearly Mendelian familial pattern of occurrence. An exception is allowed for the very rare cases with highly penetrant autosomal-dominant mutations in MAPT. The second basic criterion is that the disorder start no earlier than age 40 years. Again, cases with an MAPT mutation are an exception. The clinical onset of PSP is defined as the appearance of the first neurological, cognitive, or behavioral symptom with no likely alternative explanation that progresses in concert with other PSP symptoms. The third is that the disorder must be progressive, at least by subjective history.

The list of "basic features" proceeds to specify a long list of mandatory exclusionary criteria, 8 clinical findings, and 2 imaging findings, followed by a set of context-dependent exclusionary points. The last set is relevant only in patients with unusual features such as rapid progression, positive family history or young onset. They are designed to rule out Cretuzfeldt-Jakob disease and other prion diseases, genetic disorders and paraneoplastic and other dysimmune conditions.

Next, Table 7.5 defines 4 "domains" of PSP: ocular, postural stability, akinesia, and cognitive, each with 3 levels of certainty. Table 7.2 provides the

TABLE 7.2 Definitions of core features: Movement Disorder Society—PSP diagnostic criteria

Domain	Symbol	Feature	Definition
Ocular motor dysfunction	O1	Vertical supranuclear gaze palsy	A clear limitation of the range of voluntary gaze in the vertical more than in the horizontal plane, affecting both up- and downgaze more than expected for age; this can be overcome by activation of the vestibulo-ocular reflex; at later stages, the vestibulo-ocular reflex may be lost or the maneuver prevented by nuchal rigidity
	O2	Slow vertical saccades	Decreased velocity (and amplitude) of vertical greater than horizontal saccadic eye movements; this may be established by quantitative measurements of saccades, such as infrared oculography, or by bedside testing; gaze should be assessed by command ("Look at the wiggling finger") rather than by pursuit ("Follow my finger"), with the target >20° from the position of primary gaze; to be diagnostic, saccadic movements are slow enough for the examiner to see their movement (eye rotation), rather than just initial and final eye positions in normal subjects; a delay in saccade initiation is not considered slowing; findings are supported by slowed or absent fast components of vertical optokinetic nystagmus (ie, only the slow following component may be retained)
	O3	Frequent macro-square-wave jerks or "eyelid-opening apraxia"	Macro-square-wave jerks are rapid involuntary saccadic intrusions during fixation, displacing the eye horizontally from the primary position and returning it to the target after 200 to 300 ms; most are <1° in amplitude and rare in controls but up to 3° to 4° and more frequent (>10/minute) in PSP
			"Eyelid-opening apraxia" is an inability to voluntarily initiate eyelid opening after a period of lid closure (ie, blepharospasm); the term is enclosed in quotes because the inability to initiate eyelid opening in PSP is probably caused by overactivation of the pretarsal component of the orbicularis oculi (ie, pretarsal blepharospasm) rather than failure to activate the levator
Postural instability	P1	Repeated unprovoked falls within 3 years of onset	Spontaneous loss of balance while standing, or history of more than 1 unprovoked fall within 3 years after onset of PSP-related features

(continued)

TABLE 7.2 Definitions of core features: Movement Disorder Society—PSP diagnostic criteria (*continued*)

Domain	Symbol	Feature	Definition
	P2	Tendency to fall on the pull test within 3 years of onset	On the pull test, would fall on the pull test if not caught by examiner, within 3 years after onset of PSP-related features. The test assesses the response to a quick, forceful pull on the shoulders with the examiner standing behind the patient and the patient standing erect with eyes open and feet comfortably apart and parallel, as described in the MDS-Unified Parkinson's Disease Rating Scale (UPDRS) item 3.12
	P3	More than 2 steps backward on the pull test within 3 years of onset	On the pull test, takes more than 2 steps backward but recovers unaided, within 3 years after onset of PSP-related features
Akinesia	A1	Progressive gait freezing within 3 years of onset	Bradykinesia and rigidity with axial predominance and levodopa resistance (see red flag R1 for operationalized definition)
	A2	Parkinsonism that is akinetic-rigid, predominantly axial, and levodopa resistant	Sudden and transient motor blocks or start hesitation are predominant within 3 years after onset of PSP-related symptoms, progressive, and not responsive to levodopa; in the early disease course, akinesia may be present, but limb rigidity, tremor, and dementia are absent or mild
	A3	Parkinsonism, with tremor and/or asymmetry and/or levodopa responsiveness	Bradykinesia with rigidity and/or tremor, and/or asymmetric predominance of limbs, and/or levodopa responsiveness (see red flag R1 for operationalized definition)
Cognitive dysfunction	C1	Speech/language disorder, ie, nonfluent/ agrammatic variant of primary progressive aphasia or progressive apraxia of speech	Defined as at least 1 of the following features, which has to be persistent rather than transient: 1. Nonfluent/agrammatic variant of primary progressive aphasia (nfaPPA) or loss of grammar and/or telegraphic speech or writing 2. Progressive apraxia of speech (AOS): effortful, halting speech with inconsistent speech sound errors and distortions or slow syllabically segmented prosodic speech patterns with spared single-word comprehension, object knowledge, and word retrieval during sentence repetition (*continued*)

TABLE 7.2 Definitions of core features: Movement Disorder Society—PSP diagnostic criteria (*continued*)

Domain	Symbol	Feature	Definition
	C2	Frontal cognitive/ behavioral presentation	Defined as at least 3 of the following 5 features, which have to be persistent rather than transient:
			1. Apathy: reduced level of interest, initiative, and spontaneous activity; clearly apparent to informant or patient
			2. Bradyphrenia: slowed thinking that is clearly apparent to informant or patient
			3. Dysexecutive syndrome: eg, reverse digit span, Trails B or Stroop test, Luria sequence (at least 1.5 standard deviations below mean of age- and education-adjusted norms)
			4. Reduced phonemic verbal fluency: eg, giving words starting with a given letter (D, F, A, or S) in 1 minute (at least 1.5 standard deviations below mean of age- and education-adjusted norms)
			5. Impulsivity, disinhibition, or perseveration: eg, socially inappropriate behaviors, overstuffing the mouth when eating, motor recklessness, applause sign, palilalia, echolalia
	C3	Corticobasal syndrome	Defined as at least 1 sign each from the following 2 groups (may be asymmetric or symmetric):
			Cortical signs: (a) orobuccal or limb apraxia, (b) cortical sensory deficit, (c) alien limb phenomena (more than simple limb levitation)
			Movement disorder signs: (a) limb rigidity, (b) limb akinesia, (c) limb myoclonus
Clinical clues (optional)	CC1	Levodopa resistance	Defined as improvement of the MDS-UPDRS motor score by ≤30%. To fulfill the criterion, patients should be assessed on at least 1000 mg/d of levodopa with a DOPA decarboxylase inhibitor (if tolerated) for at least 1 month; OR once patients have received this treatment, they could be formally assessed following a challenge dose of at least 200 mg (with a DDCI)
	CC2	Hypokinetic, spastic dysarthria	Slow, low volume and pitch, harsh texture
	CC3	Dysphagia	Otherwise unexplained difficulty in swallowing severe enough to request dietary adaptations

(*continued*)

TABLE 7.2 Definitions of core features: Movement Disorder Society—PSP diagnostic criteria (*continued*)

Domain	Symbol	Feature	Definition
	CC4	Photophobia	Intolerance to visual perception of light attributed to adaptational dysfunction
Imaging findings (optional)	IF1	Predominant midbrain atrophy or hypometabolism	Atrophy or hypometabolism predominant in midbrain relative to pons, as demonstrated, eg, by MRI or [^{18}F]FDG PET
	IF2	Postsynaptic striatal dopaminergic degeneration	Postsynaptic striatal dopaminergic degeneration, as demonstrated, eg, by [^{123}I]IBZM SPECT or [^{18}F]DMFP PET

definitions of each level of each domain in more detail and adds 2 optional domains: clinical clues and imaging findings. Finally, Table 7.3 gives the combinations of features necessary to define each level of certainty for each of the PSP phenotypes.

Overall, the criteria define 16 combinations. Four "probable" combinations apply to the RS, PGF, P, and F variants; 5 "possible" combinations apply to the OM, RS, PGF, SL, and CBS variants; and 7 "suggestive" combinations apply to the OM, PI, RS, P, SL, F, and CBS variants. The literature and available additional autopsy cases were insufficient to construct robust criteria for each variant at each level. In fact, PSP-RS, the classic form, where ample literature exists, is the only variant where that was possible. For the next most common variant, PSP-P, "possible" criteria could not be formulated, leaving that form with only the highest ("probable") and lowest ("suggestive") criteria. The same is true for PSP-F. For PSP-PI, whose feature (postural instability) is part of other PSP phenotypes, only "suggestive" criteria could be formulated. For the most recently described and probably the rarest known form, cerebellar involvement in PSP (PSP-C), no criteria at all were feasible.

The MDS criteria publication also helpfully offers optional, supportive clues, including levodopa resistance, hypokinetic/spastic dysarthria, dysphagia requiring dietary adaptation, photophobia, midbrain atrophy on structural imaging, midbrain hypometabolism on functional imaging, and reduction of postsynaptic striatal dopamine receptor activity on single-photon emission computed tomography (SPECT) or positron emission tomography (PET) imaging. For this purpose, "levodopa resistance" means no response to a trial of levodopa 1000 mg/d (with carbidopa) for at least 1 month. For patients who had undergone such a trial in the past with only an unreliable or subjective result, documented absence of response to a single dose of levodopa 200 mg (with carbidopa) would suffice.

TABLE 7.3 Degrees of diagnostic certainty, obtained by combinations of clinical features: Movement Disorder Society—PSP diagnostic criteria

Diagnostic certainty	Definition	Combinations	Predominance type	Abbreviation
Definite PSP	Gold standard defining the disease entity	Neuropathological diagnosis	Any clinical presentation	def. PSP
Probable PSP	Highly specific but not very sensitive for PSP	(O1 or O2) + (P1 or P2)	PSP–Richardson syndrome	prob. PSP-RS
		(O1 or O2) + (A2 or A3)	PSP with predominant parkinsonism	prob. PSP-P
	Suitable for therapeutic and biologic studies	(O1 or O2) + A1	PSP with progressive gait freezing	prob. PSP-PGF
		(O1 or O2) + C2	PSP with predominant frontal presentation	prob. PSP-F
Possible PSP	Substantially more sensitive but less specific for PSP	O1	PSP with predominant ocular motor dysfunction	poss. PSP-OM
		O2 + P3	PSP with Richardson syndrome	poss. PSP-RS
	Suitable for descriptive epidemiologic studies and clinical care	A1	PSP with progressive gait freezing	poss. PSP-PGF
		(O1 or O2) + C1	PSP with predominant speech/language disorder	poss. PSP-SL
		(O1 or O2) + C3	PSP with predominant corticobasal syndrome	poss. PSP-CBS
Suggestive of PSP	Suggestive of PSP but not passing the threshold for possible or probable PSP	P1 or P2	PSP with predominant postural instability	s.o. PSP-PI
		O2 or O3	PSP with predominant ocular motor dysfunction	s.o. PSP-OM
		O3 + (P2 or P3)	PSP with Richardson syndrome	s.o. PSP-RS
	Suitable for early identification	(A2 or A3) + (O3, P1, P2, C1, C2, CC1, CC2, CC3, or CC4)	PSP with predominant parkinsonism	s.o. PSP-P
		C1	PSP with predominant speech/language disorder	s.o. PSP-SL
		C2 + (O3 or P3)	PSP with predominant frontal presentation	s.o. PSP-F
		C3	PSP with predominant corticobasal syndrome	s.o. PSP-CBS

Note: The basic features B1 + B2 + B3 (Table 7.2) are required for probable, possible, and suggestive criteria.

TABLE 7.4 Basic features: Movement Disorder Society—PSP diagnostic criteria

B1: Mandatory inclusion criteria	1. Sporadic occurrence[a]
	2. Age 40 years or older at onset[b] of first PSP-related symptom[c]
	3. Gradual progression of PSP-related symptoms[c]
B2: Mandatory exclusion criteria[d]	**Clinical findings**
	1. Predominant, otherwise unexplained impairment of episodic memory, suggestive of Alzheimer disease
	2. Predominant, otherwise unexplained autonomic failure, eg, orthostatic hypotension (orthostatic reduction in blood pressure after 3 minutes standing ≥30 mm Hg systolic or ≥15 mm Hg diastolic), suggestive of multiple-system atrophy or dementia with Lewy bodies
	3. Predominant, otherwise unexplained visual hallucinations or fluctuations in alertness, suggestive of dementia with Lewy bodies
	4. Predominant, otherwise unexplained multisegmental upper and lower motor neuron signs, suggestive of motor neuron disease (pure upper motor neuron signs are <u>not</u> an exclusion criterion)
	5. Sudden onset or stepwise or rapid progression of symptoms, in conjunction with corresponding imaging or laboratory findings, suggestive of vascular etiology, autoimmune encephalitis, metabolic encephalopathies, or prion disease
	6. History of encephalitis
	7. Prominent appendicular ataxia
	8. Identifiable cause of postural instability (eg, primary sensory deficit, vestibular dysfunction, severe spasticity, or lower motor neuron syndrome)
	Imaging findings
	1. Severe leukoencephalopathy, evidenced by cerebral imaging
	2. Relevant structural abnormality (eg, normal pressure or obstructive hydrocephalus; basal ganglia; diencephalic, mesencephalic, pontine, or medullary infarctions; hemorrhages; hypoxic-ischemic lesions; tumors or malformations)
B3: Context-dependent exclusion criteria[d,e]	**Imaging findings**
	1. In syndromes with sudden onset or stepwise progression, exclude stroke, cerebral autosomal dominant arteriopathy with subcortical infarcts and leukoencephalopathy (CADASIL) or severe cerebral amyloid angiopathy, evidenced by diffusion-weighted imaging (DWI), fluid-attenuated inversion recovery (FLAIR), or T2* magnetic resonance imaging (MRI)
	2. In cases with very rapid progression, exclude cortical and subcortical hyperintensities on DWI-MRI suggestive of prion disease
	Laboratory findings
	1. In patients with PSP-CBS, exclude primary Alzheimer disease pathology (typical CSF constellation [ie, both elevated total tau/phospho-tau protein and reduced β-amyloid 42] or pathological β-amyloid positron emission tomography [PET] imaging)
	2. In patients <45 years of age, exclude:
	a. Wilson disease (eg, reduced serum ceruloplasmin, reduced total serum copper, increased copper in 24-hour urine, Kayser-Fleischer corneal ring)

(continued)

      b. Niemann-Pick disease type C (eg, plasma cholestan-3β,5a,6β-triol level, filipin test on skin fibroblasts)

      c. Hypoparathyroidism

      d. Neuroacanthocytosis (eg, Bassen-Kornzweig, Levine-Critchley, McLeod disease)

      e. Neurosyphilis

3. In rapidly progressive patients, exclude:

      a. Prion disease (eg, elevated 14-3-3, neuron-specific enolase (NSE), very high total tau protein [>1200 pg/mL], or positive real-time quaking induced conversion (RT-QuIC) in cerebrospinal fluid [CSF])

      b. Paraneoplastic encephalitis (eg, anti-Ma1, Ma2 antibodies)

4. In patients with suggestive features (ie, gastrointestinal symptoms, arthralgias, fever, younger age, atypical neurological features such as myorhythmia), exclude Whipple disease (eg, *Tropheryma whipplei* DNA polymerase chain reaction [PCR] in CSF)

Genetic findings

1. *MAPT* rare variants (mutations) are not exclusionary, but their presence defines inherited as opposed to sporadic PSP.

2. *MAPT* H2 haplotype homozygosity is not exclusionary but renders the diagnosis unlikely.

3. Rare variants of *LRRK2* and *parkin* have been observed in patients with autopsy-confirmed PSP, but their causal relationship is unclear so far.

4. Known rare variants in other genes are exclusion criteria, since they may mimic aspects of PSP clinically but differ neuropathologically. These include:

      a. Non-*MAPT*-associated frontotemporal dementia (eg, *C9orf72, GRN, FUS, TARDBP, VCP, CHMP2B*)

      b. Parkinson disease (eg, *SYNJ1, GBA*)

      c. Alzheimer disease (*APP, PSEN1, PSEN2*)

      d. Niemann-Pick disease type C (*NPC1, NPC2*)

      e. Kufor-Rakeb syndrome (*ATP13A2*)

      f. Perry syndrome (*DCTN1*)

      g. Mitochondrial diseases (*POLG*, mitochondrial rare variants)

      h. Dentatorubral pallidoluysian atrophy (*ATN1*)

      i. Prion-related diseases (*PRNP*)

      j. Huntington disease (*HTT*)

      k. Spinocerebellar ataxia (*ATXN1, 2, 3, 7, 17*)

[a]*MAPT* rare variants (mutations) may lead to inherited phenocopies of the sporadic disease with a Mendelian trait pattern.

[b]*MAPT* rare variant carriers may have earlier disease onset.

[c]Consider any new-onset neurological, cognitive, or behavioral deficit that subsequently progresses during the clinical course in the absence of other identifiable causes as PSP-related symptom.

[d]Suggestive of other conditions, which may mimic aspects of PSP clinically.

[e]Need to be verified only if suggestive clinical findings are present.

TABLE 7.5 Core features: Movement Disorder Society—PSP diagnostic criteria

Level of certainty	Functional domain			
	Ocular motor	Postural instability	Akinesia	Cognitive loss
1 (most)	**O1** Vertical supranuclear gaze palsy	**P1** Repeated unprovoked falls within 3 years of onset	**A1** Progressive gait freezing within 3 years of onset	**C1** Speech/language disorder, ie, nonfluent/ agrammatic variant of primary progressive aphasia or progressive apraxia of speech
2	**O2** Slow vertical saccades	**P2** Tendency to fall on the pull test within 3 years of onset	**A2** Parkinsonism that is akinetic-rigid, predominantly axial, and levodopa resistant	**C2** Frontal cognitive/ behavioral presentation
3 (least)	**O3** Frequent macro-square-wave jerks or "eyelid opening apraxia"	**P3** More than 2 steps backward on the pull test within 3 years of onset	**A3** Parkinsonism with tremor and/or asymmetry and/or levodopa responsiveness	**C3** Corticobasal syndrome

TABLE 7.6 Supportive features: Movement Disorder Society—PSP diagnostic criteria (summary of the 2 "optional" groups of features in Table 7.4)

Clinical clues	Imaging findings
CC1: No levodopa responsiveness	IF1: Predominant midbrain atrophy or hypometabolism
CC2: Hypokinetic, spastic dysarthria	IF2: Postsynaptic striatal dopaminergic degeneration
CC3: Dysphagia	
CC4: Photophobia	

The MDS criteria await prospective autopsy confirmation. Just as important, their complexity may prove an obstacle to their widespread use outside of formal research protocols. An early report of inter-rater reliability of the MDS criteria found a kappa of only 0.64 for a diagnosis of PSP and 0.58 for the specific phenotype. (Kappa ranges from 0 to 1.0; 0.41 to 0.60 is "moderate" agreement, 0.61 to 0.80 is "substantial" and 0.81 to 1.00 is "almost perfect.") As an aside, a similar complexity-related difficulty in everyday clinical application continues to hamper use of the criteria for multiple-system atrophy published in 1998. A solution would be a computer-based data form that calculates the resulting phenotype and certainty level (Picillo et al, 2018).

Diagnosis in Early Stages 8

A large majority of people with progressive supranuclear palsy (PSP) reach medical attention for problems with balance or behavior (Maher et al, 1986). This is particularly true for the Richardson syndrome phenotype, which in pure form accounts for about half of all PSP. This chapter describes the early clinical picture of Richardson syndrome and how it may help predict the subsequent course.

At an early stage, a diagnosis of PSP may be made if the physician includes PSP on the differential diagnosis along with proximal muscle weakness, cardiac arrhythmia, transient ischemic attack (TIA), paroxysmal vertigo, paroxysmal hypotension, and epilepsy. Unfortunately, PSP does not usually make the list, even if it is formulated by a neurologist. The patient then undergoes brain magnetic resonance imaging (MRI), magnetic resonance angiography (MRA), electroencephalogram (EEG), electromyography (EMG), nerve conduction testing, electronystagmogram (ENG), Holter monitoring, echocardiogram, autonomic testing, and various blood tests. All give negative results except when an incidental abnormality leads one into more tests, each, like the original set, with its own expense, discomfort, emotional stress, physical risk, and inconvenience.

The difficulty in diagnosing PSP in the first half of the typical disease course cannot be overstated. In 1 autopsy-confirmed series, only 25% of the patients with autopsy-confirmed PSP received a diagnosis of PSP at their first clinic visit and by the last visit, the figure had risen only to 68% (Respondek et al, 2017).

There are several reasons to attempt to improve this situation. One is to save patients unnecessary diagnostic testing. Another is to allow them to enter a clinical trial for PSP. Trials may be more likely to demonstrate efficacy at an earlier stage. Furthermore, the earlier the patient starts to enjoy the benefits of a new experimental drug, the better. Even when these 2 are not relevant, patients and families find comfort in a specific diagnosis. It allows them to focus emotional energy on a known "enemy" and educational efforts on a specific condition. It allows patients and families to form supportive contacts with others with the same diagnosis and to avail themselves of the offerings of organizations devoted to PSP. Perhaps most important for those with PSP, an accurate diagnosis allows an estimate of prognosis.

The order of appearance of the various features as described here is only the most common sequence or that obtained by averaging the time to appearance of the features over a large sample of patients later diagnosed with PSP.

GAIT AND BALANCE

In about 60% of cases, the initial symptom is a fall that may or may not be blamed on an obstacle. Antecedent gait difficulty may have been attributed to aging or degenerative arthritis. Barring important injury, the first fall rarely prompts medical consultation. If the fall is backward, the family may be more likely to recognize it as pathological. A physician evaluating a patient with an unexplained fall should perform a pull test, which may provide the only positive neurological finding. Here, the examiner stands immediately behind the patient, with a wall or examining table 6 to 8 feet behind the examiner. The examiner explains that the patient will feet a tug on the shoulders and may compensate by shifting 1 leg backward but should try to keep the other leg stationary. The examiner should pull hard enough to make a healthy person of that body size have to take that single compensatory step. Immediately after delivering the pull, the examiner should shift his or her forearms under the patient's armpits to provide support if the compensatory step(s) fail. At the same time, the examiner should take a step or two backward to avoid having the patient's compensatory step(s) land on his or her own feet. The wall or exam table serves as a backup device to prevent patient and examiner from falling together in a heap. A normal result on the pull test accepts the single backward compensatory stride by 1 leg.

The search for evidence of gait difficulty early in the course requires observing the patient for a tendency to scissor, meaning crossing the legs more than necessary during gait tasks. As part of the gait exam, the patient should be asked to perform a 180-degree pivot at a prespecified point a distance away. Early gait dysfunction may take the form of an extra step during the pivot or even as a tendency to retropulse a step or 2 during the turn.

COGNITIVE AND BEHAVIORAL CHANGES

While the patient or family is unlikely to seek medical attention when the sole symptom is a few falls or mild balance difficulty, the arrival of additional symptoms may be more motivating. The most common second symptom of PSP is behavioral abnormality. It typically starts with reduced tendency to contribute to conversations unless prompted. This may be a manifestation of verbal influency, a sensitive sign of frontal lobe dysfunction, rather than any change in mood or intellect. At this stage, a test of semantic or phonemic fluency called category naming is likely to bring an abnormal result. Such a task is included in the Frontal Assessment Battery and Montreal Cognitive Assessment, 2 popular and convenient screening tests that are sensitive to frontal dysfunction. The typical task is to give the subject 1 minute to state as many words as possible within a specified category. Details of this quick and sensitive bedside test appear in Chapter 9.

Other elements of behavioral change at this early stage may include a reluctance to attend social gatherings and a loss of interest in the news of the day. In some cases, the change is in the other direction, toward disinhibited social behavior. When such a change is marked and precedes any motor issues, the possibility of frontotemporal dementia should lead the differential diagnosis. But in milder or delayed form, such change may occur in PSP. Common examples are mildly inappropriate comments to acquaintances or a tendency to grasp or handle objects unnecessarily, called "utilization behavior."

MOTOR PARKINSONISM

Mild overall bradykinesia typically also occurs at this stage, consistent with the observation that the dopaminergic substantia nigra is where the pathology of PSP starts, along with the globus pallidus interna and subthalamic nucleus. However, detecting it at this stage is usually beyond the observational acuity of the patient and family, and usually of the primary care physician as well. All of them would likely wave off the bradykinesia as normal aging.

DYSARTHRIA

The next most likely symptom to appear in the earliest stages of PSP–Richardson syndrome is dysarthria. The initial subjective report may actually be excessive vocal volume or slowing, both manifestations of spastic speech. A trained examiner at this point may also detect ataxia of speech, where the syllables are inappropriately spaced and emphasized, a phenomenon called scanning speech. (The term arises not from a flattening of vocal volume but from the opposite, the result of attempting to read a line of poetry that has been "scanned" or marked to indicate the separation of metric feet and syllabic emphasis.) A minority of patients will exhibit palilalia at an early stage, usually for single sounds or syllables but occasionally for entire multisyallabic words and even sentences. Whether this is technically a form of dysarthria, a language disturbance, or a manifestation of the behavioral disinhibition is a semantic issue.

VISUAL CHANGES

The next most common symptom at this early stage is vague visual difficulty. The patient usually reports "double vision" or "blurring." Formal refractive correction provides little or no help. The physiologic problem may be fixation instability, most commonly in the form of square-wave jerks, discussed in more detail in Chapter 10. Another common issue is slow saccades to a visual target or hypometric saccades, where the movement pauses just short of the target and then corrects. In either event, the patient fails to bring the fovea, the most sensitive part of the retina, to align with the intended target quickly enough to satisfy the perceptual demand. The problem is even more noticeable to the patient when the target is moving. The result is insufficient spatial resolution, which the patient calls "blurring." But when the patient has ample time to aim the eye at a stationary figure on a screen, as during formal refractive examination, the result is a report of normal visual acuity.

A physician examining eye movement at the early stages of PSP is likely only to detect limitation of upgaze, interpreting it as normal aging or Parkinson disease, both of which in fact include that sign in many cases. In PSP, although downgaze is the more specific abnormality, upgaze limitation often appears first and remains worse than downgaze limitation for the entire disease course.

Square-wave jerks, which eventually occur in most cases of PSP, may be present at the time of initial medical contact. They may prompt a complaint of "double vision." But examination reveals no dysconjugacy of gaze and the patient may be told that the eye exam is normal. Square-wave jerks may be detectable only by visualizing the fundus, which should be a standard part of the evaluation for any visual complaint. An examiner who has never heard of square-wave jerks may notice them if they are large and misinterpret them as lack of cooperation with the visual fixation task.

Only rarely in the early stages of PSP does the patient notice loss of saccadic gain, otherwise termed *loss of saccadic amplitude* or *gaze palsy*. In such cases, the complaint may be a reduction in the ability to see shirt buttons while dressing or the dinner plate when attempting to cut food. The family may notice the patient compensating by flexing the neck excessively during visual tasks in the lower half of space. Of course, this measure becomes increasingly difficult as the neck rigidity of PSP develops.

The clinician evaluating any undiagnosed complaint of visual difficulty should evaluate several aspects of supranuclear gaze control. One is a simple test for convergence, asking the patient to fixate on a small target brought from 18 inches to 6 inches from the nose. Note that the movement of the target should be toward the tip of the nose rather than the level of the eyes, as converging in the horizontal plane is difficult for older people and can give a false-positive result. Another sensitive supranuclear task is opticokinetic nystagmus, where the ability to generate and maintain the amplitude and rhythm of the jerks with the stripes moving up or down is impaired more than in the horizontal plane. Another is the ability voluntarily to suppress the vestibulo-ocular reflex. Here, the patient is seated on a swiveling chair with arms fully extended in front, fingers clasped as if praying, and 1 thumb protruding up. The examiner instructs the patient to maintain that position and to fix gaze on the thumb while rotating the patient slowly right and left over a 40- to 45-degree arc at a rate of about 1 full cycle in 3 or 4 seconds. The examiner observes the subject's eyes throughout. In the healthy state, they remain stationary in their orbits, but in patients with disorders of supranuclear gaze control, the successive passage of objects in the room through the patient's visual field produces jerk nystagmus.

EYELID CHANGES

The eyelids may also show motor abnormalities very early in the course of PSP (Golbe et al, 1989; Yoon 2005). Lid retraction and reduced blink rate combine to produce a wide-eyed stare. In some patients, the dystonia of the facial muscles produces not only the general facial overinnervated appearance reminiscent of a reaction to a bad odor but also excessive blinking. Bright light may precipitate or aggravate the blinking and may even produce an unpleasant sensation for the patient, in which case we apply the term *photophobia*. Some patients first notice this when viewing a brightly spotlighted area in an otherwise dark theater. Ophthalmologic evaluation without close attention to vertical saccadic eye movement will typically diagnose the problem as conjunctival irritation, which may in fact be present at this stage because of dryness caused by reduced eyeblink, called exposure keratopathy.

DYSPHAGIA

The next most frequent early symptom is dysphagia for liquids with a need to sip slowly or to clear residua with a cough. The patient and family are unlikely to report that issue to the physician unless specifically prompted. Even then, the patient and family may not have acknowledged the abnormality, and the physician will be none the wiser without having the patient drink a cup of water in the examining room. Difficulty with solids is not a common issue for patients with PSP until the middle disease stages. An exception is the patient whose frontal lobe–related motor disinhibition includes a tendency to overload the mouth.

OLFACTION

Smell identification tests and olfactory perception threshold testing are abnormal in Parkinson disease (PD), dementia with Lewy bodies, and Alzheimer disease. In PSP, results vary from normal to a point about halfway between those and controls (Krismer et al, 2017; Doty et al, 1993). Olfaction in multiple-system atrophy is slightly better than in PSP, but the difference is insufficient for clinical diagnostic use.

CSF AND BLOOD MARKERS

Neurofilament light chain (NfL) in both plasma and cerebrospinal fluid (CSF) is elevated in atypical parkinsonisms, including PSP, corticobasal degeneration, multiple-system atrophy, frontotemporal dementia, and dementia with Lewy bodies, as well as in amyotrophic lateral sclerosis and traumatic brain injury (Hansson et al, 2017). However, it is not elevated in PD, probably because the source of that protein, large myelinated axons, are relatively spared by the pathology of PD (Jabbari et al, 2017). But it cannot differentiate PSP from the other non-PD conditions, limiting its utility as a diagnostic trait marker. The plasma NfL level correlates with PSP disease severity as measured by the PSP Rating Scale in cross-sectional series (Rojas et al, 2016). There is also unpublished evidence that the level rises with disease progression in individual patients, rendering serum NfL potentially useful as a convenient, noninvasive state biomarker. More recently, the ratio of NfL to phospho-tau in CSF has been found to track the PSP Rating Scale closely, at least over the 1-year period of observation during a drug study. Furthermore, that ratio at baseline predicted the rate of progression over the ensuing year (Rojas et al, 2018).

So serum NfL and CSF NfL/p-tau are promising candidates, along with MRI morphometrics, as replacements for the PSP Rating Scale as a primary outcome measure in neuroprotective clinical trials. However appealing this may be for neuroscientists, regulatory agencies still prefer outcome measures based on the clinical examination and assessment of disability in daily activities, and this trend is, if anything, growing. However, "surrogate markers" for disease severity in PSP have an important role in understanding treatment physiology and, to the extent that they predict future clinical events, in clinical care and as trial outcome markers as well.

Cognitive and Behavioral Features 9

Many behavioral neurologists claim progressive supranuclear palsy (PSP) as one of their own. Although PSP is traditionally considered a "parkinsonism," implying that its motor features predominate, in fact as many as 40% of cases referred to movement disorder centers start with behavioral abnormalities. In series gathered by behavioral neurologists, that fraction is of course far higher. Some experts even consider PSP to be no more than a segment of the spectrum of frontotemporal dementia (FTD). That spectrum includes 3 behavior-predominant conditions (behavioral-variant FTD, semantic dementia, and progressive nonfluent aphasia) and 3 motor-predominant conditions (corticobasal degeneration, FTD–amyotrophic lateral sclerosis, and PSP).

"SUBCORTICAL DEMENTIA"

PSP is the archetype of *subcortical dementias*, a term that has been discredited but still appears in the literature (Albert et al, 1974). With the archetype of vascular dementia or Parkinson disease (PD), such patients display slowing of thought with apathy, depression, and impaired abstraction. It contrasts with *cortical dementia*, typified by Alzheimer disease and featuring amnesia, agnosia, apraxia, and aphasia. More recently, the 2 categories have been found to overlap clinically and anatomically too often to be useful. Modern imaging techniques prompt a reclassification of most patients with "subcortical dementia" into a new category called "frontal system dementia." One excellent study (Pillon et al, 1991) further classified the subcortical dementias into 3 categories: a frontal type typified by PSP, a type with difficulty in concentration and data

acquisition typified by Huntington disease, and a combination of these, typified by PD.

VARIABILITY AND PITFALLS

The dementia of PSP is highly variable with regard to the mix of specific cognitive deficits and their order of onset relative to the motor features (Brown
et al, 2010). Some series find no more than minimal cognitive impairment that
does not affect daily activities, especially when tests requiring visual scanning
are avoided or controlled for statistically (Kimura et al, 1981). Of the patients
with early onset of "dementia," most of the deficits are behavioral rather than
cognitive. Most prominent here is apathy, with depression and pseudobulbar
affect less so. The first 2 of these can easily give the family and physician an
impression of dementia. A very common initial observation by the family is
withdrawal from social situations. Together with slowness of response termed
bradyphrenia and difficulties in visual fixation during conversation, the apathy
of PSP can easily create or exaggerate the impression of dementia. Another common diagnostic error is assuming that the neuropsychiatric features such as
apathy and depression always are part of the degenerative disorder. They
may, instead, be a reaction to the dementia or motor disability or an adverse
effect of medication such as anticholinergics or dopaminergics. Yet another
common error is diagnosing the early behavioral features of PSP as a primary
psychiatric disorder such as agitated depression or bipolar disorder and treating
with neuroleptics, only to precipitate severe parkinsonian motor deficits.

FEATURES OF PSP DEMENTIA

When true cognitive impairment does begin, it usually features problems with
visual fixation and attention, verbal fluency, and inhibition of motor behavior.
These features typically remain the worst cognitive problems in PSP and distinguish the dementia of PSP from that of PD, Huntington disease, and Alzheimer
disease, even after controlling for overall dementia severity (Pillon et al,
1991).

The visual fixation difficulty often causes the gaze to remain fixed on the
examiner. When asked to regard a different target, the head will turn but the
eyes remain on the original target. Other patients will maintain fixation on an
inconsequential object in the room and remain unable to shift the gaze to the
examiner, even during direct conversation. In fact, impairment in shifting attention has been found to be more impaired relative to other frontal lobe functions in PSP than in PD or multiple-system atrophy (Robbins et al, 1994).

The first signs of verbal nonfluency may be a paucity of spontaneous speech, word-finding problems, and echolalia, a tendency to repeat others' phrases. The last of these is an example of the stimulus-linked nature of many cognitive deficits in PSP. A sensitive test for verbal fluency is asking the patient to say as many words as possible within a given phonemic category in 1 minute. The words cannot be numbers or proper nouns and must be semantically independent (e.g., "run" and "runner" are counted as 1). The category may be such things as the initial letter or items found in a supermarket. The initial letters F and S allow the English-speaking patient perhaps greatest opportunity to list taboo words, demonstrating evidence for disinhibition. The popular Montreal Cognitive Assessment and more specialized Frontal Assessment Battery impose 11 words in 1 minute as the lower bound of normal for this task.

A popular bedside test of motor disinhibition in PSP is the "applause sign" (Dubois et al, 2005). The examiner instructs the patient to observe and imitate, then claps his or her hands 3 times over a period of 2 or 3 seconds. An inability on the part of the patient to inhibit the action after 3 claps correlated well with the presence of PSP in 1 study, correctly identifying 81.8% of the patients in the comparison of PSP and FTD and 75% of the patients in the comparison of PSP and PD (Dubois et al, 2005).

Likewise, other disinhibited behavior of PSP is often linked to a stimulus. Patients who cannot arise from a chair on request may nevertheless do so very quickly after catching sight of a desired object out of reach, even one across the room. This phenomenon, unsympathetically called the "rocket sign," is a common cause of injury in PSP. Other chair-bound patients may quickly stand when a table is moved away from their chair or a lap belt unfastened. Caregivers must be made aware of this phenomenon.

Other frontal cognitive tasks on which patients with PSP perform disproportionately poorly relative to their overall degree of dementia are in describing similarities, imitation of hand gestures, attention to a multistep task, spatial planning, and accuracy of problem solving (Pillon et al, 1991; Robbins et al, 1994).

An odd, possibly frontal, behavior in a minority of patients with PSP is involuntary groaning. Its volume ranges from a soft, intermittent, cat-like purr to a fully phonated roar that interferes with the family's conversation except for the few seconds required for the patient to take a breath or to speak. I know of no clearly effective treatment. The groaning is suppressible for brief periods, like tics, prompting me to try alpha-2 agonists such as clonidine and guanfacine. These sometimes succeed, although their superiority to placebo is a question. Of course, dopamine blockers, the most effective treatment for typical tics, are contraindicated in PSP and other degenerative parkinsonisms.

The Mattis Dementia Rating Scale is used widely in research trials and clinical care and is sensitive to frontal dysfunction. In a drug trial, the largest observational series on PSP dementia to date, 311 patients with PSP scored lowest in the subsection on initiation/perseveration, where 73% performed below the lower limit of normal. They did somewhat better in the other 4 subscales comprising memory (33%), conceptualization (24%), construction (20%), and attention (14%). Only 20% of patients with PSP showed no significant impairment on any cognitive domain, and 39% showed impairment restricted to a single domain.

CORTICAL PROBLEMS IN PSP

Rare or absent in PSP are anomic aphasia and difficulty in word or sentence comprehension. However, the disorder does impair sentence completion as well as category fluency, as mentioned above. This same sort of aphasia is common to other frontal lobe disorders. A rare initial presentation of autopsy-proven PSP is primary progressive aphasia (Boeve et al, 2003), where the motor features start years after the language problem. The most frequent pathology underlying primary progressive aphasia is that of frontotemporal dementia, not PSP.

Apraxia in PSP can involve eyelid opening, discussed in more detail in the chapter on eye movement (Chapter 10). PSP also displays apraxia of eye movement and of speech, both similarly misnamed, where the initial difficulty is overcome on the second or third try.

The clearest example of apraxia in PSP, however, is in the limbs. This clinical overlap with corticobasal degeneration can produce diagnostic difficulty. Apraxia and dystonia are the 2 motor features of PSP that can in a few cases be highly asymmetric, as in corticobasal degeneration (CBD). The rare occurrence of asymmetric apraxia (typically with dystonia) as the presenting sign of PSP has been called the "corticobasal syndrome onset" of PSP (Josephs et al, 2006). However, apraxia in PSP is usually symmetric. It is most commonly of the ideomotor type, where the patient has difficulty producing a complex hand movement on verbal request (Bruns et al, 2013). The apraxia of PSP involves both transitive ("hammer a nail," "throw a ball") and intransitive ("wave goodbye," "hitch-hike") ideomotor tasks and consistently impairs constructional tasks such as copying geometric figures (Pharr et al, 2001).

NATURAL HISTORY OF DEMENTIA IN PSP

The 1991 study of Pillon et al, which remains one of the best on this topic, defined dementia as a score exceeding 2 standard deviations (SD) from the mean of control subjects given the same battery of tests. In that cross section of 45 patients at all stages of PSP, 26 (58%) satisfied this criterion for dementia. Twenty-four of the patients with PSP had serial evaluations, the first of which was performed a mean (SD) of 2.7 (0.3) years after symptom onset. At that point, 9 patients (37.5%) were demented. After an average of 4 years of disease, the last formal evaluation in that study, 70% were demented. Another study showed that even a year after onset, over half of all patients displayed some degree of frontal cognitive loss (Litvan et al, 1996).

NEUROPSYCHIATRIC DEFICITS

Apathy is defined as indifference, even to one's illness. Depression, on the other hand, emphasizes an alteration of mood and in some cases produces apathy. The PSP literature often fails to distinguish between the two. Another shortcoming of many of the published surveys is the absence of a subject group with Alzheimer disease (AD) for comparison with a more familiar primary dementing illness. The sole study to date that avoided both drawbacks evaluated 22 consecutive patients with PSP and 50 with AD using a formal neuropsychiatric scale (Litvan et al, 1996). Ninety-one percent of the patients with PSP had apathy and 36% reported disinhibition, both figures higher than for AD. Lower figures for PSP relative to AD were reported for depression, anxiety, and agitation, and none had hallucinations or delusions.

Only 2 studies to date have compared PSP with PD with regard to neuro-psychiatric signs. One (Menza et al, 1995) relied on unstructured psychiatric evaluation and did not attempt to control for group differences in age, disease duration, and overall disability. It found more disinhibition and pseudobulbar affect in PSP but no differences otherwise. It did not specifically mention apathy. The other study (Aarsland et al, 2001) did control for some of the demographic differences mentioned, but the 103 patients with PD were from a community epidemiologic study in Norway and the 61 with PD from a tertiary referral clinic in the United States. It found the same results as the other study plus more hallucinations and delusions in the PD group. The authors concede the possibility that the greater prevalence of psychosis in PD could be explained by those patients' greater reliance on dopaminergic treatment or by possible admixture of some cases of dementia with Lewy bodies.

Apathy, despite receiving short shrift in much of the PSP literature, in fact is the most common nonmotor feature of the disease. It was present in 62% of a cross section of patients with PSP in 1 study, with severe apathy present in 8%. A study from China (Ou et al, 2016) found apathy in all 27 of their patients with PSP (and in 11% of controls) despite an average PSP duration of only

3.6 years. Patients may deliberately disguise their apathy during an office visit, and if the performance is normal as tested by brief, routine tests of cognition such as orientation and memory, the physician may dismiss the family's report that the patient is behaviorally disabled. The PSP Rating Scale's item on "withdrawal" queries the caregiver on any loss of social interaction in an attempt to reveal apathy. On the PSP–Quality of Life questionnaire, 3 of the 45 items directly or indirectly assess apathy.

We must conclude that further study, probably using modern functional imaging, is needed to adequately understand the neuropsychiatric features of PSP and their anatomic underpinnings (Josephs et al, 2011; Whitwell et al, 2011).

Eye Movement 10

EARLY FEATURES

Naming the disease for its gaze impairment was perhaps an unfortunate choice. Most physicians have not heard of progressive supranuclear palsy (PSP), and even among those who have, a majority seems to know only that it involves motor parkinsonism and vertical gaze impairment. Even then, most will not recognize the gaze loss until it reduces the amplitude of vertical pursuit movement, which occurs a median of nearly 4 years after onset of the first symptom. By that time, the patient and family may have undergone rounds of fruitless diagnostic procedures and therapeutic trials, not to mention endured the stress conveyed by their physicians' puzzled expressions.

Patients with early PSP vary in their subjective visual complaints. Only rarely will the patient perceive and report difficulty moving the eyes. A subtle defect in maintaining fixation on a target, or in accurately moving to a new target, will prevent the patient from using the fovea, where the density of rods is greatest. This will cause a loss of spatial resolution, prompting a complaint of "blurring." The patient may perceive an image at 1 or more stops along the path of a multistep saccade, prompting the complaint of "double vision." The same complaint may arise from the less common situation where the eyes are affected asymmetrically.

ANATOMY

The pathology responsible for the gaze palsy of PSP affects much of the brainstem. Vertical saccades are initiated by excitatory burst neurons in the rostral interstitial nucleus of the medial longitudinal fasciculus, located just rostral to the third nerve nucleus, and are maintained by tonically firing neurons in the interstitial nucleus of Cajal, also in the midbrain. Horizontal saccades are initiated in the paramedian pontine reticular formation and maintained by the medial vestibular nucleus and nucleus prepositus hypoglossi, both in the medulla. Assisting the process of initiating saccades are neurons in the reticular formation of the medulla that relax the antagonist eye muscle. Maintaining the eyes at rest when no saccade is desired are "omnipause" neurons in the nucleus of the raphe interpositus in the pons. All of these degenerate in PSP, and the list involves multiple neurotransmitter systems. This is why the ocular motor pathways may prove the most resistant to treatment of the various brain systems involved in PSP.

SACCADIC PHYSIOLOGY

The first PSP-specific, objective finding in most cases is slowing of downward saccades without limitation of range of gaze. In severe cases, the eye moves so slowly and smoothly as to prompt the description, "marble-in-oil phenomenon." As a practical matter for the clinician, saccadic slowing can be defined as a movement that the examiner can see progressing from one point to another, while the progression of normal-velocity saccades is seen by the examiner only as 2 stationary positions. For large saccades, peak velocity is 500 degrees per second, so a saccade between the position of primary gaze and a target at the periphery of normal gaze, which is 50 degrees away, will occupy only 100 ms. This is too fast for the examiner's visual system to process.

While downgaze palsy is more specific for PSP, upgaze limitation in saccadic amplitude is more common. A typical series found limitation of upgaze alone in 47%, both upward and downward in 30%, and pure downward in only 23%.

As the lids typically will cover the eyes during downgaze, it is usually necessary for the examiner to start the exam by having the patient lower the lids, then to gently place thumbs on the lids and raise them while instructing the patient to allow that. Then have the patient fixate on a fixed target such as the examiner's nose and command, "look down," "nose," "look up," "nose," "right," "nose," "left," "nose." Asking the patient to follow a moving target will not accomplish the task because it is insensitive to mild or even moderate gaze impairment.

The initial vertical saccadic slowing is most likely to start with difficulty returning to the position of primary gaze from the up or down position. Patients who follow the instruction not to move the head for the initial eye movement will typically move the head to assist in the return to primary gaze. This is a tipoff for the examiner, who should then repeat the procedure after instructing the patient to keep the head stationary throughout. Another tipoff is the "around-the-houses sign," where an attempt at vertical gaze produces an eccentrically curved movement that may or may not reach the target.

Shortening of saccades, prompting a corrective movement, is another early sign. Such hypometric saccades may shorten enough to produce what is informally and inaccurately called a "saccadic movement," proceeding in steps throughout its course. A better term is *multistep saccade*.

GAZE APRAXIA

A common abnormality in PSP that can interfere with testing of saccades is gaze apraxia. This sign may also occur very early in the disease course but often in subtle form. The patient hears and understands the gaze command but cannot initiate the saccade at first. The difficulty often resolves after multiple repetitions of the command or a chance to follow a moving target. This phenomenon may be confused with "visual grasping," which can also interfere with gaze testing and is probably a result of frontal lobe damage, an analog of manual grasping or verbal perseveration. Here, the patient maintains fixation on an object of intrinsic interest such as a face despite commands to direct the gaze elsewhere. The examiner can avoid it by substituting a finger or pen as the target.

SUPPLEMENTARY MANEUVERS

Other maneuvers may reveal subtle vertical saccadic impairment. One is opticokinetic nystagmus (OKN). A variety of tools can be used, from a rotating drum striped in the direction of the axis of rotation to a strip of cloth with wide stripes perpendicular to its long axis. The examiner should practice on healthy subjects to learn how fast to move the stripes to elicit consistently crisp nystagmoid movement as the subject counts the stripes as they move past a fixed point of gaze. In PSP, some stripes may be missed or the nystagmus is irregular because the velocity of the saccade returning to find the next stripe is too slow for the task. Other defects in cortical eye fields or brainstem structures integrating the reflex may also impair OKN. The key in PSP is that OKN in the vertical plane is impaired far more than in the horizontal plane. While it is an early sign in PSP, the same abnormality in less severe form can occur in Parkinson disease (PD).

Another sensitive sign of early vertical gaze palsy is curved diagonal saccades. A variant of the "around-the-houses sign" described above, this is where the examiner places his or her two hands at the periphery of the patient's visual fields, at the ends of an axis tilted 45 degrees from the vertical. The patient is instructed to move gaze from one to the other in turn on command. The patient with early vertical gaze palsy will launch the saccade along more of a horizontal direction, correcting the course partway through the movement.

A sign that appears relatively early and consistently is square-wave jerks, termed *Gegenrücke* in the earlier literature. These occur during attempts to fixate on a stationary target and may be observed more easily during fixation on a light held at least a meter away in a darkened room, with a second light illuminating the eye. When they are of low amplitude, they are best seen on funduscopic exam. The jerks are conjugate (ie, both eyes moving in parallel), horizontal, and 0.5 to 3.0 degrees in amplitude. Each jerk starts at the primary position of gaze fixation and pauses for about 200 ms at the end of its movement before the eyes return to their original, primary fixation point. The jerks are irregular in their frequency, which ranges up to 4 per second. In some patients, they may be as infrequent as every few seconds. They cannot be voluntarily suppressed by the patient (Troost, 1992).

Limitation of upward saccades is common in PD and in normal aging. But after a typical interval of 2 to 4 years after the initial motor onset in PSP–Richardson syndrome (PSP-RS), there is consistent limitation of the amplitude of downward saccades. Reflex saccades, as during passive head tilt during visual fixation, the vertical oculocephalic or "vertical doll's eyes" maneuver, remain normal until very late in the disease course and, in many patients, are never lost. This becomes difficult to test in more advanced patients because of axial rigidity.

Horizontal saccades are affected after the problems in the vertical directions are well established. A very early sign is loss of the ability to voluntarily suppress vestibulo-ocular reflex. The patient sits in a swiveling chair with arms extended in front, hands clasped, and 1 thumb extended upward. The patient is instructed to keep the head and arms still with respect to the body and to maintain visual fixation on the thumb while the chair is slowly rotated right and left while the examiner observes the eyes. In PSP and some other conditions, opticokinetic nystagmus is produced by objects in the room passing through the visual field, but healthy persons are able to suppress it by fixating on the thumb, which is not moving with respect to themselves. Further details on this test appear in Chapter 8.

Loss of convergence is another nonspecific sign of loss of gaze control in the horizontal plane. It should be tested by moving the visual target toward the tip of the patient's nose and observing for loss of convergent fixation before the target reaches a point 18 inches away.

"Cogwheel pursuit," hypometric saccades, and saccadic slowing occur initially, followed by reduction in gaze amplitude and finally by complete ocular fixation in every plane except for large square-wave jerks. At this stage, horizontal oculocephalic reflex movement may remain to some extent, but as more brainstem integrative areas and the third, fourth, and sixth nerve nuclei themselves become involved in the disease process, even these responses disappear.

EYELID ABNORMALITIES

The classic image of a person with PSP includes a wide-eyed stare. Lid retraction is the result of impaired inhibition of sympathetic innervation to Müller's muscle. Reduced blink rate common in PSP and can produce disabling conjunctival drying. Blink rates in PSP typically average 5 per minute, less than the 10 to 15 for PD and 20 to 25 for healthy elders (Golbe et al, 1989). There is conjunctival drying with reactive lacrymation, but access to the oily secretions of the Meibomian glands during waking hours is insufficient to maintain conjunctival integrity.

Blepharospasm is a form of focal dystonia that occurs in a quarter of patients and is as common in early stages as later. It starts as frequent blinking, often with photophobia. The latter may be triggered not only by diffuse illumination but also sometimes by intense, local illumination, as in a spotlighted area in a dark theater. The patient struggles to open the lids using the frontalis muscles and then resorts to using the fingers. Sometimes this only intensifies the orbicularis oculi contraction. The result is functional blindness, at least for periods of several minutes or hours. The most efficacious treatment we have for any aspect of PSP at present is injection of botulinum toxin into orbicularis oculi. Details of injection sites, techniques, and toxin dosages are beyond the scope of this volume. The potential complication is ptosis resulting from diffusion of the toxin to the levator palpebrae superioris or Müller's muscle.

The term *apraxia of lid opening* has been used to refer to the blepharospasm of PSP and other conditions in situations where there is no visible corrugation of the orbicularis oculi. But the term *apraxia* supposes an intact subcortical motor system, clearly not the case in PSP. Furthermore, the contraction conforms to the electrophysiological features of dystonia and the absence of correlation with other forms of apraxia in PSP (Chen et al, 2010; Grandas. 1994). The appearance of apraxia is mimicked by the intermittency of the contraction and by its susceptibility to emotional relaxation.

Apraxia of lid closing is another misnomer, but this is a form of loss of supranuclear control of lid closing rather than a form of dystonia. Patients with PSP may be unable to close the lids on command despite a normal-appearing blink and unable to keep the lids closed, even gently, despite repeated commands from the examiner.

DIAGNOSTIC ALTERNATIVES

Conditions other than PSP can cause supranuclear vertical gaze palsy disproportionate to any abnormality in the horizontal plane (Sequeira et al, 2017). Among neurodegenerative disorders, corticobasal degeneration, multiple-system atrophy, and dementia with Lewy bodies are the most common PSP mimics. A few patients with amyotrophic lateral sclerosis can have upgaze restriction. Spinocerebellar ataxia type 2 features horizontal saccadic slowing, but vertical movement are spared.

The same is true for Gaucher disease type 3. Niemann-Pick type C features vertical gaze palsy in a majority of cases and should be considered the leading diagnostic possibility when a PSP-like condition develops before age 40 years.

Paraneoplastic encephalitides related to anti-Ma2 antibodies feature vertical gaze palsy, usually upward, in a majority of cases, and if left untreated in the later stages or if treatment fails, some develop other eye movement phenomena and even can lose all saccadic function. Parkinsonism and other basal ganglia phenomena may also occur on a paraneoplastic basis. Treatable with immunomodulatory agents and removal of the inciting neoplasm, a paraneoplastic cause should be sought by anti-Ma/Ta antibody testing in patients with a rapidly progressive PSP-like picture.

Antibodies against glutamic acid decarboxylase (GAD) produce a chronic encephalitis featuring multiple eye movement abnormalities as well as stiff-person syndrome or cerebellar ataxia. A recently described condition associated with antibodies against IgLON5 produces a PSP-RS phenotype in 22% of cases (Gaig et al, 2017).

Whipple disease is often cited as a potential PSP mimic, but my own informal survey of PSP referral centers worldwide reveals no such cases within living memory. While Whipple disease may cause vertical gaze palsy progressing to complete ophthalmoplegia, postural instability, cognitive deficits, and dystonia, its other features are not features of PSP. These include oculomasticatory myorhythmia (where rhythmic convergent eye movement occurs simultaneously with masseter contractions), prominent ataxia, myoclonus, seizures, fever, arthralgias, and prominent gastrointestinal symptoms.

Perhaps also in the category of infection mimicking PSP is Creutzfeldt-Jakob disease (CJD), where vertical gaze palsy may occur early or late in the course. Other common features of CJD are parkinsonism and postural instability. Patients with a very rapidly progressive PSP phenotype should therefore receive magnetic resonance imaging with attention to the diffusion images in search of gray matter signal abnormalities, electroencephalography, and usually lumbar puncture.

Vertical gaze palsy may result from masses dorsal to the midbrain such as pineal tumors, gliomas, or metastases. Late-life decompensation of chronic congenital hydrocephalus may do the same.

Dysarthria 11

NATURAL HISTORY

Dysarthria appears in the first year of symptoms in 70% to 80% of patients with progressive supranuclear palsy (PSP). Its median time to appearance after disease onset, as measured by patient and family report, is 40 months, and speech becomes unintelligible, as measured by that item in the Unified Parkinsonism Disease Rating Scale, at a median of 71 months after symptom onset (Sonies, 1992).

FEATURES

The speech in PSP typically has a strained, harsh, even growling quality. Its speed is usually slow, and volume is highly variable, even within a sentence, in contrast to the consistently soft, rapid, monotonic dysarthria of Parkinson disease (PD). This is called "spastic" speech, although that term leads one to expect a larger set of pyramidal signs, which are usually absent in PSP. The dysarthria of PSP also features slurred articulatory errors, stuttering, palilalia, and ataxia. In fact, a study of 44 patients using a classification system for dysarthria that rates the contributions of spastic, ataxic, and hypokinetic components found that all patients with PSP displayed spasticity plus at least 1 of the other 2 elements. All 3 types were present in 64%. This despite an average disease duration in those patients of only 2.4 years (Kluin et al, 1993). A smaller formal assessment of abnormal speech characteristics using a different nosologic system in 22 patients at a variety of disease stages found the most common issue to be slurring, at 50%, followed by reduced sustained phonation, reduced volume, hypernasality, and slowed rate (Sonies, 1992).

MANAGEMENT

Only 1 study has evaluated rehabilitation therapy for dysarthria in PSP. Sale et al (2015) assessed the Lee Silverman Voice Treatment (LSVT Loud), a standardized, copyrighted protocol developed by Ramig et al (2001) for dysarthria of PD. The technique attempts to enhance vocal cord control, to use enhanced phonation and air movement as a trigger to improve articulation, and to retrain the patient's sensory monitoring of vocal output as a feedback technique.

The study was small, with only 16 patients with PSP, and did not include a control group receiving traditional speech therapy or no therapy. It did include an internal standard comprising 23 patients with PD, a condition in which the intervention had already proven useful. The PSP group's mean PSP Rating Scale score was 41, with an average disease duration of 4 years, a point a few months after a diagnosis is first made in a majority of patients. The treatment was delivered in 16 one-hour, one-on-one sessions over 4 weeks.

Both the PSP and PD groups showed statistically significant improvements in the range of frequencies produced and in the vocal volume during a reading task. There was no improvement in a sentence repetition task or in the maximum volume during spontaneous speech. Nor was there a follow-up to determine the persistence of improvement. We must conclude that no speech therapy protocol has proven to be efficacious for PSP but that LSVT Loud has preliminary, uncontrolled data that merit further investigation in PSP.

Some patients can learn to use a word pointing device such as one in a computer tablet application. However, by the time the dysarthria requires this, the dementia, loss of manual dexterity and downgaze difficulty conspire to make the device impractical. Still the speech evaluation should include consideration of such a device in any patient with PSP.

A major issue is whether the dementia of PSP allows the patient to practice techniques taught during therapy sessions and to monitor their benefit. As a practical matter, I focus rehabilitation efforts for my patients with PSP on swallowing and gait, the 2 areas where complications can be life-threatening. If the patient or caregiver asks about speech therapy, I explain the paucity of efficacy data and I assess the travel logistics, insurance coverage, caregiver availability, and, perhaps most important, the caregiver's and patient's expectations based on what they have heard from others. This is one of many areas of PSP care where providing hope can be most valuable.

Dysphagia 12

Considering the importance of dysphagia in progressive supranuclear palsy (PSP), the paucity of published literature on the topic is surprising and dismaying.

NATURAL HISTORY

The median time from initial symptom of PSP to onset of dysphagia is around 4 years, and 9% of patients complain of dysphagia as one of the initial symptoms, but these figures derive from patients' and families' subjective, often retrospective reports (Nath et al, 2003; Golbe et al, 1988). Patients whose dysphagia develops within the first 2 years of PSP onset have an age–adjusted mortality ratio of 3.91 ($P < .01$), a measure of their risk of dying over any subsequent unit of time relative to patients without that risk factor. For patients with dysphagia developing after the 2-year point, the ratio was only 1.6, which was not statistically significant (Nath et al, 2003).

NORMAL AND ABNORMAL PHYSIOLOGY

The normal process of swallowing starts with voluntary oral manipulation of the food bolus during chewing followed by transfer of the bolus to the pharynx. In this phase, dysphagia may result from dysfunction of any part of the central or peripheral motor system. The most common defect in the oral phase in PSP is delayed initiation of swallow, present in 84% of a cross section of patients (Sonies, 1992; Litvan et al, 1997). Close behind are disorganized or hyperkinetic movement of the tongue, slowing of the oral phase, and impaired bolus transfer to the pharynx. Less common are abnormalities in movement of the velum. A few patients exhibit fragmentation of the food bolus, which may be a result of repeated, involuntary swallows analogous to the motor perseveration seen in other motor and language tasks in PSP.

Next is the pharyngeal phase, where brainstem reflexes predominate over voluntary control of movement. At its start, the soft palate elevates to protect against nasopharyngeal reflux, an action rarely if ever impaired in PSP despite the common finding on exam of reduced palatal elevation during phonation. At that point, the bolus reaches the faucial arches and the hypopharynx. Then the hyoid bone elevates, causing the epiglottis to descend and the larynx to elevate. The result is closure of the airway. During this phase, the deficits, occurring in nearly all patients with PSP, are vallecular pooling and uncontrolled falling of a food bolus into the pharynx. Less frequent are pooling in a piriform sinus, unilateral bolus transport, and incomplete emptying of the pharynx into the esophagus.

The time required by healthy persons for the oral and pharyngeal phases of a swallow of 10 cc of pureed solid is only 1 to 2 seconds, but the average for PSP is 4 seconds, and even then it may be incomplete.

The esophageal phase consists of involuntary peristalsis. About half of patients with PSP exhibit delayed peristalsis, and a quarter have esophageal-pharyngeal reflux. An important difficulty in PSP is difficulty producing an adequate cough to clear food that has refluxed or has pooled in valleculae or pyriform sinuses.

The dysphagia of PSP only occasionally exhibits silent aspiration, in contrast to that of advanced Parkinson disease (PD). In fact, awareness of dysphagia is far more common among dysphagic patients with PSP than in those with PD. Choking or the urge to cough is far more common in PSP than in PD despite the greater impairment of brainstem reflexes in PSP. Rigidity of the tongue is rare in PSP, while it is common in PD, analogous to rigidity of the limbs in the 2 disorders.

The first symptom of dysphagia is typically coughing on thin liquids that have penetrated past the glottis and into the larynx (Goetz et al, 2003; Muller et al, 2001). However, other difficulties described above may appear on the modified barium swallow before a complaint of dysphagia for liquids.

MANAGEMENT

A formal swallowing evaluation should occur when any symptom of dysphagia appears. This may take the form of coughing on thin liquids; the need to avoid certain dry, tough, or leafy solids; difficulty eating foods with a variety of textures such as vegetable soup; slow swallowing; or the need to have food cut small. A common early feature of PSP is the tendency to overload the mouth, an expression of motor disinhibition resulting from frontal lobe impairment. This can cause what might be called *secondary dysphagia*.

The evaluation should be performed by a speech-language pathologist (SLP), who examines the lips, mouth, and pharynx and may have the patient eat or drink sample foods. The evaluation should also include a formal radiographic modified barium swallow (MBS), which may have to be ordered specifically but is ordinarily scheduled to be performed immediately after the SLP's history and physical examination regardless of its results. The MBS is a cineradiograph performed while the patient consumes a range of foods and liquids mixed or impregnated with radiopaque dye. The imaging is performed both laterally and anteroposteriorly, although the first is far more useful in this setting. The radiologist reports the progress of the bolus through at least the oral and pharyngeal phases and part of the esophageal phase, reporting such abnormal phenomena as slowing of oral transfer, fragmentation of the bolus, nasal regurgitation, vallecular or pyriform sinus pooling, glottis penetration, and frank aspiration. If coughing is observed, its efficiency at clearing the offending matter is reported.

In the setting of PSP, imaging of the full length of the esophagus during food ingestion, an unmodified "barium swallow," is not ordinarily useful unless reflux is reported.

There are no studies evaluating indications for performing a swallow evaluation/MBS in patients with PSP. But given the importance of aspiration in the morbidity and mortality of the disorder, it seems prudent to order the evaluation at the first observed or reported sign of dysphagia for liquids or solids or when the patient has difficulty managing secretions. At this point, while awaiting the swallow evaluation/MBS, the clinician should advise that pending the formal advice, patients with dysphagia for thin liquids should avoid such beverages in favor of thicker ones such as fruit nectars. The same can be accomplished by mixing a starch-based thickening agent into thin beverages. This measure can even be used with water, although the slight taste of the thickener may require masking by a beverage with a more intense flavor of its own. The patient or family may ask about use of a straw or have already instituted one. This causes the liquid to enter the mouth at increased velocity and may aggravate the dysphagia.

For patients with dysphagia for solids, the caregiver has usually found and instituted any needed interim measures such as avoiding dry or fibrous solids. Still, the MBS will be as valuable a guide here as it is with liquids.

Ordinarily, the SLP reviews with the patient and caregiver the results of the evaluation, including the MBS, and issues a list of recommendations for modifying the diet or eating technique. The SLP should counsel the patient and caregiver to allow them to understand, accept, and implement the advice. The clinician ordering the evaluation should receive a copy of the recommendations and, at the next visit, inquire into their implementation and efficacy. Patients and caregiver may take the recommendations more seriously after such follow-up and reinforcement. The clinician ordering the evaluation should also instruct the caregiver to call should the SLP's counseling seem insufficient.

Unfortunately, levodopa is no more efficacious against the dysphagia of PSP than in any other area. A study of 18 patients treated with levodopa showed improvement in only 2 patients as assessed by fiber-optic endoscopy (Warnecke et al, 2010).

FEEDING TUBE PLACEMENT

The decision to place a percutaneous endoscopic gastrostomy (PEG) is a difficult one in PSP and one with little or no literature as a guide. In practice, patients' and families' desire to prolong life is usually overpowered by the emotional aversion to the obvious and, some would say, dehumanizing, mechanical form of daily life support in a severely immobile and demented loved one (Goldberg et al, 2014).

An analysis of disability milestones in PSP found that among patients who had received a feeding gastrostomy, the procedure was performed a median of 87 months after symptom onset, with death arriving an average of 6 months later.

Traditional indications for PEG placement are 1 episode of aspiration pneumonia, prolongation of meals to the point of interfering with operation of the household, weight loss from malnutrition, or coughing on every swallow. However, by the time a patient with PSP has reached one of those milestones, dementia has in most cases impaired the quality of life to the point that the family is likely to choose to "let nature take its course." If dementia is not severe at the time the dysphagia prompts consideration of a PEG, most patients and families will opt for the procedure, even if the motor deficits are severely impairing the quality of life. Severe pain, as from traumatic complications or decubiti, may produce exceptions to that rule.

The dilemma as to PEG placement may be compounded by the occasional experience of improvement in dysphagia and other deficits in PSP after PEG placement as a result of improved nutrition. This may allow clamping of the tube and return to oral feeding after proper dysphagia reevaluation. As for PEG in any medical setting, patients and families must be advised that PEG will not reduce the risk of aspiration from oral secretions or esophageal reflux.

An advance directive, if available, serves as a valuable guide to a patient's wishes with regard to PEG placement, although it is not legally binding. Patients who are maximally immobile and mute but not severely demented should be consulted on the matter even if an advance directive exists. Teaching the patient small finger movements to convey "yes" or "no" allows the patient's current wishes to be known. Of course, this should be preceded by a careful explanation of the procedure and its implications at a level consistent with the patient's education and degree of dementia. Adequate time over several days must be given to the patient to consider, especially as impulsive decisions are a common feature in PSP, even in its early stages. In cases with little risk of aspirating small amounts of ice cream or other treats ("recreational eating"), the decision to place a PEG may be easier.

PALLIATIVE MEASURES

A full discussion of management of patients with terminal disease that includes dysphagia is beyond the scope of this volume. However, it must be said here that a suction machine at the bedside can be a major help. The caregiver and perhaps even the patient can learn to use it to remove oral secretions. It provides a measure of dignity in its prevention of sialorrhea and may delay the risk of aspiration, although data for this are not available. This machine may form part of a hospital-like room, often set up in the family's living room to allow the patient to avoid stairs, provide room for an overnight hired aide, and allow the family undisturbed sleep upstairs. Such is the degree to which care for a loved one with advanced PSP can come to dominate the life of the family.

Physical and Occupational Therapy 13

Progressive supranuclear palsy (PSP) presents some challenges to physical and occupational therapists that may not apply to other neurological conditions. This chapter, consistent with the rest of this book, will not attempt to teach physical therapists (PTs) and occupational therapists (OTs) the standard care of patients with immobility and dementia but will highlight the special needs and solutions for those with PSP.

GOALS

The first task of the PT and OT is to provide education on the motor aspects of PSP, a disease that the patient and family probably had never heard of until the physician said, "It's PSP. Here's a prescription for PT. Bye." Put more charitably, physicians are notoriously hurried and may lack the ability or inclination to explain things at the level appropriate to the listener. Typically, the patient will differ from the caregiver in cognitive skills and, in the case of an adult child caregiver, in educational attainment. This means that the explanation received from the physician may have been pitched to one level, leaving the other either underinformed or confused.

The next task is to train the caregiver. The most common example may be techniques for assisting the patient in arising from a chair and returning there safely. This can be especially difficult for patients with severe axial rigidity, as occurs in PSP. As for any motor disorder, the task of arising from a chair will be eased by starting with the feet placed close to the chair. But rather than lifting the patient by the upper arm, which may stress the patient's shoulder joint and the caregiver's back, the caregiver can take advantage of the axial rigidity of PSP by applying a forward horizontal pull to the back of the neck. When the patient's center of gravity is over the feet, the patient will then be able to supply the upward force needed to reach a standing position. For a right-handed caregiver, this is best accomplished by standing in front of the patient, a little to the patient's left, facing the patient at an angle. This removes some stress on the caregiver's back, relying on the legs to supply most of the power to pull the patient's upper body forward. For more disabled patients or for those with kyphosis rather than the typical upright posture of PSP, it may help to use one's left hand to grasp both of the patient's hands to help pull the trunk forward as the caregiver's right hand supplies additional forward force to the back of the neck.

OBSTACLES

The social withdrawal and apathy that are very common in PSP make it difficult in many cases to convince the patient to maintain social interactions. The PT and OT sessions may offer the patient's only regular interactions with anyone other than the caregiver. Use this opportunity to stimulate and reinforce the patient's social performance rather than sticking strictly to "business." Encouraging the patient to join group exercise activities is an important way to leverage the limited time available with the PT/OT.

The frontal lobe pathology of PSP makes patients uninventive in finding workarounds and in anticipating and avoiding risks. Furthermore, the same frontal deficits include disinhibition, especially when it comes to gait and balance challenges. The patient with PSP may abruptly arise from the chair and attempt to walk across the room to retrieve something, only to fall after 1 or 2 steps. They readily acknowledge that the action was risky but say that they just needed to retrieve that item. The issue, then, is not ignorance of their disabilities but inability to anticipate consequences or to take precautions. This contrasts with the patient with Parkinson disease, in whom appropriate or excessive caution is the rule.

The PT should advise the patient to scan the environment before arising from the chair and once standing to tilt the head down to compensate for poor downgaze. Neck flexion may be as difficult as downgaze in patients with PSP, given the nuchal rigidity and even retrocollis that occurs in a few patients.

Additional insight into falls in PSP is provided by Lindemann et al (2010), who showed that falling frequency in those patients is not correlated with rigidity or bradykinesia but with measures of brainstem function on the PSP Rating Scale and with a measure of distractability in a dual-task situation. Presentation of a cognitive task as a distractor caused the stride to shorten and the cadence (steps per minute) to increase and become irregular. This suggests that care-givers and other cohabitants of patients with PSP should be advised not to attempt to speak unnecessarily with the patient during gait.

GAIT RETRAINING AND ASSISTIVE DEVICES

In gait retraining, the patient should be taught to avoid scissoring, especially on turns. This means turning the feet in the new direction and allowing the body to follow. The analogous advice applies to teaching use of a walker dur-ing turns. Canes are problematic in patients with PSP because the falls are typi-cally backward and because canes are too easy to forget to use. I therefore do not recommend a cane at any point for patients with PSP. Rather, I prescribe a PT evaluation as soon as gait difficulty appears and tell the patient that I expect that the PT will recommend a walker.

Traditional frame walkers are typically too light to prevent falls in PSP, but they are easily folded and lifted into the car's trunk by a small, elderly caregiver. It may therefore be useful to keep such a walker for outings where the care-giver will remain at the patient's side to provide contact guarding. However, the principal walker for use at home should be heavier and have swiveling wheels at the front with nonswiveling wheels at the back. The "Rollator" style, with brakes and a seat, often works well for patients with PSP. It seems not to matter whether the hand brakes are active, as on a bicycle, or passive, where the brake handles must be continuously squeezed to keep the brakes disengaged. The latter design is useful in preventing the walker from rolling away from the user during transfers but requires constant hand flexion during use. A seat with some form of backrest is useful, but the patient must wait for assistance before letting go of the handles, turning, and sitting. Patients with PSP tend not to be that cau-tious, and caregivers should be taught to use great care in allowing the patient to undertake this maneuver.

The "U-Step II" walker is often a good option for those with PSP, as it pro-vides a bit more stability against lateral falls by virtue of its U-shaped frame in a plane a few inches off the ground. It has a low center of gravity, and its shape allows the user to remain close to the walker's "footprint." It offers an optional mechanical resistance to backward falls, assuming the user continues to grip the handles. Like some other walkers, it can be equipped with a laser project-ing a line on the floor across the user's path as a visual stimulus to overcome gait freezing. However, many patients with PSP may not be able to gaze down-ward to use it. It also has an audible electronic clicking feature to allow the user to pace steps at the desired frequency, but the utility of this feature in PSP is not clear. The U-Step's drawbacks start with its greater weight, 22 pounds, compared with 15 to 19 pounds for conventional 4-wheel walkers with brakes. Its brakes offer only a passive configuration, and its relatively small, 4-inch front wheels (compared with 6- or 8-inch front wheels in other models) may present a problem with uneven outdoor surfaces. The U-Step allows the user to step on the back end of either arm of the U frame to lift the front of the walker over an obstacle. Again, the ability of patients with PSP to use this feature is a question and possibly a safety issue. The U-Step is far more expensive, typically over $500, compared with a typical walker's price of $150.

HOME ADAPTATIONS

Adaptations of the home environment to the downgaze and balance deficits are important. Coffee tables, loose rugs, and grandchildren's toys are a risk for those with PSP. Grab bars should be installed not only at the toilet and shower but at all points of the patient's usual path around the home. It is critical to clear a path around the home for the walker lest the patient become discouraged and decide that using the device is not worth the bother.

EXERCISE

To complement fall prevention training, patients should be taught to perform exercises to improve strength and aerobic conditioning. A stationary bike seems to be useful, as long as the caregiver is present to assist in mounting and dismounting. In the PT department, treadmill training with physical support has been shown anecdotally to be useful (Suteerawattananon et al, 2002). A 2018 review of the 12 published reports of rehabilitation efforts comprising a total of 88 patients with PSP demonstrated modest benefit in balance and in fall reduction. However, most of the reported experience was not controlled or randomized, the duration of benefit was not usually reported, and the types of interventions varied widely (Intiso et al, 2018).

GAZE RETRAINING

PT and OT measures also include retraining the patient's ability to perform tasks requiring vertical gaze(Di Fabio et al, 2007; Zampieri et al, 2009; Zampieri et al, 2006). This may include exercises in reading signs placed at varying heights on a wall. Large-print books are easier for those with difficulty moving the eyes accurately from the end of 1 line down to the start of the next. The patient may also be trained to better direct the gaze at the dinner plate by teaching the habit to first fixate on the fork held at eye level and then slowly to lower it to the plate. This takes advantage of the persistence of pursuit gaze in PSP after volitional gaze is lost. Another solution to the dinner plate problem is to place the plate on a platform atop the table.

Caregivers of male patients with PSP will almost unanimously agree that misaiming of the urinary stream is a problem, although they never raise that issue spontaneously. Apathy and dementia play roles here as well, of course. The solution is to convince the patient that sitting on the toilet is the best option for voiding.

Gaze retraining has also been used as a route to gait and balance retraining. Zampieri and Di Fabio (2008) have studied the ability of gaze retraining to improve balance. They compared conventional balance retraining to a paradigm where patients with PSP received the same training along with a computer-assisted saccade exercise, a saccadic task with auditory feedback and an exercise in eye-foot coordination. They found that the dually trained group improved significantly in time required to stand up and in gait speed, while 3 other measures showed no change and the balance-only group actually did better in 1 measure. The patients receiving the visual training also showed improvements in saccadic measures.

Palliative Care 14

The words, "sorry, there's nothing I can do for your PSP" should never escape the specialist's lips, and even in the end stages, care should not be relegated to the primary care physician alone. The neurologist and other specialists and ancillary medical professions will be valuable sources of advice in easing discomfort and preventing further complications. This is an especially important point for a disease as complex as progressive supranuclear palsy (PSP) (O'Sullivan et al, 2008; Uitti et al, 1999).

This chapter will not attempt to describe the clinical care of all the possible deficits in late-stage PSP. That appears in the specific chapters devoted to those disease features and in the chapter on drug treatment (Chapter 18). Nor will this chapter discuss details of the many and complex aspects of care for patients with advanced immobility, dysphagia, and dementia. Rather, here I provide an overview and general guidance in caring for such patients.

First, a semantic point. In a sense, all care in PSP is palliative, as there is still no specific treatment for the underlying disease process, and any intervention only serves to ease the symptoms. But "palliative care" is often confused with "end-of-life care." In PSP, the latter should be reserved for the last 6 to 12 months of life, after the PSP Rating Scale has reached the 60s or 70s. In fact, this time horizon is the criterion commonly used by hospice programs.

In rendering end-of-life care, the clinician should acknowledge the patient's specific symptoms as they are reported. This not only prompts formation of a care plan but also provides a form of self-respect for the patient and caregiver. The ability of the patient to report symptoms at that stage will be impaired by dementia, depression, and/or apathy. These phenomena will also reduce the motivation of the family to provide care. A bit of teaching may mitigate this unfortunate situation.

A new medical specialty, palliative care, has arisen recently. Such physicians typically work at cancer centers, where their services are a routine and accepted part of care. They may have valuable contributions to the care of end-stage PSP as well, but the neurologist should be careful not to abandon the patient at the time of such a referral. The palliative care specialist will be particularly useful in diagnosing and managing depression, in counseling patients facing death, in managing any pain (although this affects only a minority in PSP), in supervising hospice services, and in counseling families attempting to make difficult and emotionally fraught decisions.

It will be apparent to anyone reading the rest of this book that "palliative care" becomes relevant even in the first stages after a diagnosis of PSP (Bukki et al, 2014). According to the American Society of Clinical Oncology, palliative care is appropriate for patients who have limited ability to care for themselves; who have not received, no longer receive, or are unlikely to receive benefit from specific treatment; and who are not eligible to participate in a clinical trial. These conditions apply to most patients with PSP, even in the first few years of illness. In PSP, there is no "honeymoon period" analogous to the first 5 years of Parkinson disease (PD).

The stress on the caregiver should also factor into the clinician's management. One recent study (Schmotz et al, 2017) found that caregivers of persons with PSP reported more signs of depression and worse scores on a caregiver burden inventory than those of persons with PD with similar levels of disability. Furthermore, the caregiver burden became severe even in the early stages of PSP. A study looking at the patient-caregiver relationship in PSP from another angle assessed patients' views on what constitutes quality of life (Fegg et al, 2014). They listed the quality of their relationships with family and friends and leisure activities as more important than their neurological health. Similarly, compared with healthy controls, patients with PSP cited leisure activities with their caregivers and other relatives and friends as more important than health status as determinants of their quality of life, while the opposite was true for the controls (Schrag et al, 2003). The lesson should be obvious for physicians whose view of the care of persons with PSP starts and ends with the writing of prescriptions.

PAIN

Relief of pain is traditionally the physician's first duty. In 1 cross-sectional study, pain described by patient and/or caregiver as at least "slight" was present in

25% of patients with PSP and in 89% of those with PD (Kass-Iliyya et al, 2005). Its severity was far less in PSP than in PD. The location of the pain also differed. In PD, 20% of the pain was located in the torso and head, while that was never the case in PSP in that series, where it was always in the limbs, followed by neck and shoulders. None of the PSP pain met criteria for neuropathic pain, while this did occur in 33% with PD. Pain improved on levodopa in 25% with PSP and 57% with PD, but this was not compared with placebo. One report found that intractable pain in the nuchal muscles caused by the retrocollis of PSP responded to intravenous lidocaine, a routine part of the armamentarium in pain clinics (Schlesinger et al, 2009). However, pain is rarely so severe as that in PSP and is usually manageable using acetaminophen or nonsteroidal anti-inflammatory drugs. Alternatives are daily gabapentin, pregabalin, and amitriptyline, although the last drug may sometimes aggravate the postural instability in PSP. Acupuncture, massage, and joint mobilization by a physical therapist are also recommended (Wiblin et al, 2017). None of these options has been evaluated by a randomized trial.

Sleep 15

A MULTIFACTORIAL PROBLEM IN PSP

Nocturnal insomnia and daytime hypersomnia have long been studied in progressive supranuclear palsy (PSP) but their importance to patients' quality of life has been well recognized only recently (Abbott, 1992; Aldrich, 1992). In PSP, the sleep problem is compounded by urinary urgency, where a nighttime awakening is often accompanied by an effort to reach the bathroom, a trip made treacherous by the postural instability, visual difficulty, and impulsivity of PSP. The situation is aggravated by the likelihood that the caregiver who usually provides gait assistance may remain asleep. Yet at the neurologist's visit, the time constraint, the apathy of PSP and the press of more urgent symptoms typically push sleep issues off the agenda. This is one reason I included an item on sleep in the PSP Rating Scale. It not only asks about difficulty falling asleep and staying asleep but also asks the patient or caregiver to estimate whether the total sleep per average night exceeds 5 hours. There is no expectation that this will be an accurate quantification of sleep but that the reply may reflect subjective satisfaction with sleep performance.

Depression and dementia are common in PSP, but the sleep disturbances are common even in their absence. Nevertheless, total sleep time in PSP declines in parallel with scores on the Mini-Mental Status Exam. Sleep-related symptoms, or family reports, in PSP center on not only difficulty achieving sleep and frequent nocturnal awakenings but also a sensation of tension or inability to find a comfortable position at bedtime. Changing position is difficult or impossible and the early morning awakenings are often followed by an hour of remaining awake in bed.

VENTILATORY PROBLEMS

The prevalence of sleep-disordered breathing in PSP ranges from 0% to 55% in various studies and in any case is far from specific to that disease. Sleep apnea in PSP may be obstructive, central, or mixed type and may occur in any sleep stage. It is not often severe, but it may contribute to daytime somnolence, and patients with PSP who have that symptom to a troubling degree, especially in combination with loud snoring, should be referred to a sleep clinic for an evaluation and polysomnogram. However, experience suggests that patients with PSP have even more difficulty than others complying with continuous positive airway pressure masks during sleep, possibly because of their dementia and impulsivity.

REM AND REM BEHAVIORAL DISORDER

The cardinal abnormality on polysomnography in PSP is reduction in rapid eye movement (REM) sleep, and what remains shows a disordered electroencephalogram (EEG) with abnormal slowing and absence of normal sawtooth waves. These abnormalities are sufficiently sensitive and specific for PSP to serve as a differential diagnostic tool, and they do progress in severity over time. Ultimately, there may be no sleep at all some nights. Sleep latency (the time required to fall asleep) is prolonged. Sleep efficiency (the fraction of the night spent sleeping) is only 43% in PSP, lower than the 63% for Parkinson disease (PD), and the periods of sleep are highly fragmented, with little slow-wave sleep and REM sleep.

Reduction in REM sleep is disproportionate to the reduction in total sleep time. The latency to REM onset after sleep commences is highly variable, on both sides of the normal mean. Slow waves and alpha rhythm appear commonly during REM sleep, and the normal sawtooth waves gradually disappear over the disease course.

REM behavioral disorder (RBD) is not rare in PSP and the other tauopathies, contrary to published allegation, occurring in 35% of patients with PSP. This compares to 95% for PD, where it is useful as a predictive diagnostic feature years before any motor symptoms appear. Eye movements during REM sleep lose velocity and amplitude; their vertical movement is more severely affected than horizontal, and they eventually disappear entirely. This, of course, parallels the changes in voluntary saccades during wakefulness. In the early stages, rapid eye movements may occur during non-REM (NREM) sleep stages. It is important for the clinician to distinguish RBD from nocturnal confusion, which is common in PSP. Clonazepam, one of the first-line treatments for RBD, can aggravate nocturnal confusion. Polysomnography may aid in this differentiation. It is not clear whether melatonin, which can also ameliorate RBD, carries the same risk, but personal experience suggests not.

OTHER CHANGES IN SLEEP PHYSIOLOGY

In parallel with the loss of REM sleep in PSP, stage 1 sleep is increased from the 10% that is typical in the healthy elderly to 35% of total sleep. Stages 3 and 4 are similarly increased, albeit highly fragmented. Sleep spindles lose amplitude, and their component waves slow from the normal 12–14 Hz to 10–11 Hz. The spindles become less frequent as the disease progresses and eventually disappear. The K-complexes of stage 2 sleep become similarly disordered and rare. An unusual pattern called "alpha-delta sleep" develops during NREM sleep, with intrusions of 8- to 9-Hz activity along with diffuse, irregular slow waves. None of these abnormalities is common or severe in Parkinson disease. In depression, eye movements during REM sleep become more frequent, the opposite of what occurs in PSP.

In some cases, these changes make it difficult to distinguish REM and NREM sleep from each other and a waking from a sleep EEG in a patient with advanced PSP.

The prevalence of restless leg syndrome (RLS) in PSP is a matter of some disagreement, ranging from 4%, which is no different from controls, to 52%. A typical figure for PD is 10%. The responsiveness of RLS in PSP to the usual remedies such as dopaminergics and opiates is not known.

DAYTIME SLEEPINESS

True daytime sleepiness is also increased in PSP, but narcolepsy is rare, contrasting with PD, dementia with Lewy bodies, and multiple-system atrophy (MSA). Despite poor nocturnal sleep, true daytime naps, as opposed to a report of sleepiness, are relatively uncommon in PSP. A consistently hyperaroused state therefore is a fair characterization (Walsh et al, 2017). Daytime hypersomnia in PSP can culminate in advanced cases into a constant state of poor arousability but with eyelids open and no loss of postural tone in the wheelchair. In that moribund state, the EEG shows a continuous mixed-frequency pattern that does not vary over the course of the day or night.

In MSA, the range of abnormalities seen in PSP may occur, but in milder form, and nocturnal insomnia is less severe.

PATHOGENESIS

The pathogenic basis of disordered sleep in PSP follows neatly from the disease's anatomic distribution (Hauw et al, 2011). The pontine tegmental nuclei (especially the pedunculopontine tegmental nucleus), the reticular and intralaminar nuclei of the thalamus, raphe nuclei, locus ceruleus, nigrostriatal pathway, and periaqueductal gray are all relatively consistently involved in the pathology of PSP. Orexin-producing cells of the hypothalamus are also affected (Yasui et al, 2006). Loss of nigral neurons contributes importantly to daytime somnolence because dopaminergic tone supports wakefulness.

Imaging 16

Of all the categories of diagnostic markers for progressive supranuclear palsy (PSP), imaging procedures hold the greatest near-term promise, both as a "trait" marker to establish a diagnosis and as a "state" marker to quantify the degeneration (Whitwell et al, 2017).

Per the general approach of this book, imaging modalities still far from clinical utility will not be discussed in detail. Rather, the discussion will center on the current standard of clinical practice and on what that standard may become in the near future. It will also describe currently used imaging modalities that are important outcome measures in clinical trials in PSP, even if they are not (yet) used as primary outcome measures.

GENERAL COMMENTS

First, a few issues:

The first step in the clinical evaluation of a new imaging technique as a trait marker (a qualitative test as opposed to a quantitative test of disease severity) must be in a group of subjects who have already been diagnosed via accepted clinical criteria. But if that study gives positive results, the imaging technique must then be evaluated in subjects who do not already meet diagnostic criteria, that is, subjects who mimic the "real world" of early stage or diagnostically equivocal individuals. Classifying those subjects as PSP or non-PSP would then require some "gold-standard" diagnostic technique. At present, for PSP, this means either autopsy or observation over time with repeated application of validated clinical diagnostic criteria.

In evaluating an imaging technique, comparing PSP to healthy controls is a start, but it's not enough. To mimic the "real world" of the movement disorders clinic requires comparisons with disorders in the differential diagnosis of PSP. These comprise corticobasal degeneration, the parkinsonian form of multiple-system atrophy (MSA), dementia with Lewy bodies, vascular states, frontotemporal dementia, and Alzheimer disease. Furthermore, the prevalence of these disorders in the subject group should reflect their prevalence in the population.

For trait markers, diagnostic accuracy is assessed by calculating the area under the receiver operating characteristic curve (AUC). The vertical axis is sensitivity, the horizontal axis is 1 minus specificity, and each axis ranges from 0 to 1.0. An acceptable marker's AUC should be at least 0.8 when the comparison group reflects a real-world clinic population. This typically translates into sensitivity and specificity of at least 80% each. As for any diagnostic test, maximizing sensitivity is important when measuring the burden of disease in a population, as for a medical economic study or a prevalence survey. Specificity is more important when it's critical to exclude non-PSP from a group such as one undergoing a treatment trial or observational study.

Early phase studies of candidate markers between subject groups may only show a separation of mean values. Such comparison, however statistically significant it may be, is not an adequate validation of a marker intended for clinical use at the individual level. However, in comparing response to treatment between subject groups, comparison of means would usually be valid. Nevertheless, the better a state marker performs in an AUC calculation, the more useful it will be in this setting.

For state markers, the measure should correlate with disease severity as measured in a diverse cross section of individuals with the disease. The "gold standard" against which the candidate marker is compared must be accepted and validated, albeit expensive, unwieldy and/or, risky. Furthermore, the state marker should be able to measure disease progression over time in individual patients, a particularly important issue in PSP. In practice, few markers in neurodegenerative diseases show a smooth progression over time in every individual, and one must be satisfied with a smooth progression of the mean values for a group followed longitudinally. This is adequate for clinical trials in using large subject groups.

The recently described "minority phenotypes" of PSP have barely been studied with regard to imaging. Nearly all studies of PSP diagnostic markers to date have used inclusion criteria designed to identify the classic PSP–Richardson syndrome (PSP-RS). This may allow validation of the imaging modality for PSP-RS but not necessarily for a PSP variant where a different anatomical emphasis may produce a very different imaging abnormality or no abnormality at all.

MAGNETIC RESONANCE IMAGING: MORPHOMETRY

First, it is important to remember that focal atrophy on magnetic resonance imaging (MRI) reflects the clinical syndrome, not necessarily the underlying pathology. For example, corticobasal degeneration of the PSP type (CBD–Richardson syndrome) can display the same low midbrain/pons ratio as PSP-RS. This limits the utility of morphometric MRI as a stand-alone diagnostic trait marker.

The pathological process in PSP starts in the globus pallidus internus, the subthalamic nucleus, and the substantia nigra. As these structures are small and not adjacent to cerebrospinal fluid (CSF) spaces, changes in their chemical and anatomical structure are too subtle to serve as an early diagnostic marker on currently available anatomic imaging. Although emerging functional imaging techniques hold great promise, clinical practice continues to depend on anatomic imaging using conventional MRI.

Radiologic diagnosis of PSP began in the 1980s, when computed tomography (CT) in the axial plane showed atrophy of the midbrain worse than the pons, atrophy of the thalami causing disproportionate widening of the posterior third ventricle, and atrophy of the frontal and temporal lobes causing disproportionate widening of the anterior Sylvian fissure (Figure 16.1a and 16.1b)

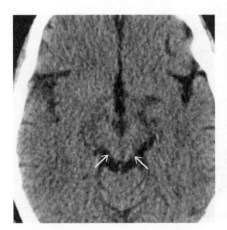

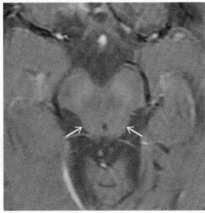

FIGURE 16.1A CT scan showing moderate atrophy of the dorsal midbrain in a patient age 68 years with PSP for 4 years and a PSPRS score of 45.

FIGURE 16.1B Normal T1 MRI axial cut showing a convex surface of the dorsal midbrain (arrows).

(Schonfeld et al, 1987). Problems were the poor resolution of CT scanning for small structures, variability in scanning angles, and artifact in imaging posterior fossa structures because of interference from the dense bone of the skull base. Still, routine CT can provide an initial hint that PSP, at least in its moderate to advanced stages, belongs on the patient's differential diagnosis.

The field leapt forward with the advent of MRI, which revealed the same areas of atrophy more reliably and quantitatively, and where subtle parenchymal signal characteristics could now be observed. The famous "hummingbird sign" or "penguin sign" of PSP arises from atrophy of the midbrain in midsagittal images without proportionate atrophy of the pons (Figures 16.2 through 16.4). The result is a sleek "head" and plump "body." The "Mickey Mouse sign," equally famous, arises from atrophy of the midbrain peduncles on axial sections, causing the normal rectangular shape to become rounded, with atrophy disproportionate dorsally, giving the peduncles a circular shape. The "morning glory sign," less famous, is caused by atrophy of the dorsal midbrain, making its lateral margins flat or concave in axial cuts rather than convex (Figure 16.5).

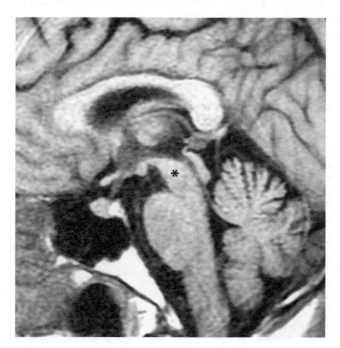

FIGURE 16.2 Midsagittal T1 MRI section from a 62-year-old patient 2 years after first her first symptom of PSP, a fall. PSPRS score of 21. The midbrain is minimally atrophic but still within normal limits.

* midbrain

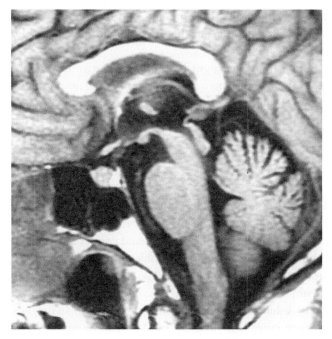

FIGURE 16.3 The same patient 2 years and 3 months later, with PSPRS score of 41. There is now a clear, but still moderate, hummingbird sign with atrophic midbrain and normal pons.

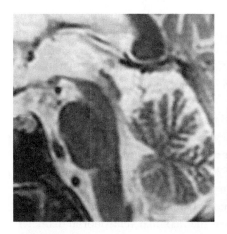

FIGURE 16.4 Advanced hummingbird sign in an 82-year-old man with PSP for 7 years and a PSPRS score of 72.

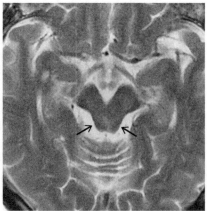

FIGURE 16.5 The upper midbrain on axial section performed with the image in Figure 16.4. The dorsal portion of the midbrain now has nearly straight lateral margins, termed the "morning glory sign."

The result vaguely resembles the profile of a morning glory blossom, with the midbrain peduncles analogous to the distal parts of the smoothly diverging petals.

These whimsically named signs have no quantitative definitions, however, and can be obscured by variations in patient positioning or scanning angles. The hummingbird sign can be obscured by slight departure from a precise midsagittal cut position. This may allow the "midline" cut to include some of the peduncle, increasing the apparent anteroposterior diameter of the midbrain.

THE MIDBRAIN: PONS RATIO

An extra level of detail is justified for this section, as for the section on clinical diagnostic criteria, because of its central importance in the everyday diagnosis of PSP. As there is still no definitively final and correct information for either task, each clinician facing a diagnostic problem involving PSP must gain a feel for the issues rather than applying a "cookbook" approach that a guide for the clinician's coat pocket might provide.

Limiting the value of assessments of midbrain atrophy in diagnosing PSP is that the same structure also atrophies in MSA-parkinsonism (MSA-P), a frequent PSP clinical mimic in its early stages. However, the MRI in MSA-P and the other forms of MSA also typically displays marked atrophy of the pons and cerebellum, structures that atrophy only slightly in PSP. Indeed, the ratio of the diameter of the dorsal midbrain to the diameter of the belly of the pons as measured in the midsagittal plane has been proposed as a diagnostic differentiator (Massey et al, 2013), using a cut point of 0.52 (Figure 16.6). This result was confirmed by Owens et al (2016), who found 100% specificity of this cut point for PSP against a cohort with MSA and Parkinson disease (PD). In 82% of the patients in whom the sign occurred, it preceded the clinical diagnosis of PSP by a mean of 15 months.

It is easy to measure the midbrain and pontine diameters on an existing MRI image using the linear measurement device in the display software or a traditional ruler on a screen or printout. For this reason, the midbrain/pons anteroposterior (AP) diameter ratio of 0.52 is presently the most widely used radiographic criterion for the midbrain atrophy of PSP. For each structure, a line is drawn at the maximal rostrocaudal diameter, and another line is constructed perpendicular to the first, across the maximal ventrodorsal diameter. The diameter of the midbrain does not include the aqueduct or the collicular plate, and the diameter of the pons does not include its tegmentum. The ventrodorsal measurements are the ones used in the calculation (Massey et al, 2013).

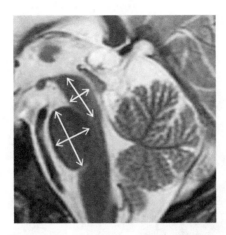

FIGURE 16.6 In this 60-year-old woman with corticobasal syndrome, the midbrain and pons are normal in their ventro-dorsal (antero-posterior) diameters: midbrain 1.1 cm, pons 1.6 cm. The diameters are drawn per Massey et al (2013). Ovals are constructed to cover the midbrain and pons, excluding the tectum for each. The diameter is the length of the line perpendicular to the long axis of each. The long (rostro-caudal) diameters are shown here only to indicate the positioning of the short (ventro-dorsal) diameters. Massey et al found the ratio of diameters of MB/P of < 0.52 or a midbrain absolute diameter of < 9.35 mm to each have 100% specificity for PSP. The absolute diameter measurement has 90% sensitivity for PSP in a clinically diagnosable stage. Earlier stages are often normal for both measures.

However, a ventrodorsal diameter does not take into account atrophy in the rostrocaudal dimension. Nor does it take account of atrophy of the midbrain tectum, where a slight departure from a midsagittal position, in addition to spoiling the hummingbird sign as described above, will exaggerate the size of the tectum by including a greater diameter of the colliculi, placed just right and left of the midline.

To address the first of these drawbacks in the midbrain/pons diameter ratio, Oba et al (2005) developed the midbrain/pons area ratio. It uses a midsagittal image of a 3- to 4-mm thickness. It separates midbrain from pons on a line from the ventral brain surface at the superior pontine notch to the dorsum of the midbrain at the level of the caudal extent of the quadrigeminal plate, where it meets the superior medullary velum. It separates pons from medulla by a line from the inferior pontine notch running dorsally, parallel to the first line (Figure 16.7). The area of the midbrain is drawn to exclude the aqueduct, quadrigeminal plate, and mammillary bodies. The last appears on the midsagittal image as a teardrop hanging from the rostral tip of the midbrain and is actually the partially volumed medial portions of both mammillary bodies.

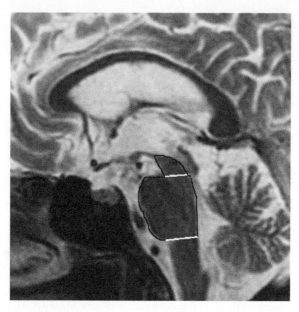

FIGURE 16.7 Areas of the midbrain (MB) and pons (P) to be used in calculating the magnetic resonance parkinsonism index (MRPI). The line between midbrain and pons is drawn from the superior pontine notch to the caudal end of the tectum. The line at the caudal end of the pons is drawn parallel to the first line, starting at the inferior pontine notch. Both areas exclude the tectum. MRI viewing software can often automatically calculate the areas of manually drawn figures.

Oba et al (2005) found no overlap between the midbrain area/pons area ratio between their 21 subjects with PSP and their comparison groups of 23 with PD, 25 with MSA-P, and 31 controls. The means (ranges) were as follows: PSP, 0.124 (0.09–0.15); PD, 0.208 (0.17–0.30); MSA-P, 0.266 (0.18–0.49); and controls, 0.236 (0.18–0.32). It can be measured with the region–of–interest outlining tool available on many imaging display software systems supplied by radiologists on the compact disk along with the images. As it can be difficult to control the cursor in outlining the midbrain and pons, it is best to enlarge the image as much as possible and to measure the areas several times and to average the values before calculating the ratio.

When MSA-P is a diagnostic consideration, a more sensitive and specific marker of PSP on MRI is the magnetic resonance parkinsonism index (MRPI). It uses areas of pons and midbrain as above but combines it with measurements of the superior and middle cerebellar peduncles. Its formula is (pons area / midbrain area) × (middle cerebellar peduncle width / superior cerebellar peduncle width) or (P / M) × (MCP / SCP).

In PSP, the MRPI exceeds 13.55. In the seminal series of Quattrone et al (2008), this value fully separated subjects with PSP from those with PD, MSA-P, and healthy controls. The MRPI has particular value in distinguishing PSP from PD, where the sensitivity was found by Nigro et al (2017) to be 100% and the specificity 99%. The added value of the MRPI relative to the pons/midbrain in distinguishing PSP from MSA-P comes from the fact that in MSA-P, the MCP atrophies markedly and the SCP atrophies only moderately, while in PSP, the MCP atrophies minimally and the SCP atrophies moderately.

The midbrain and pontine areas are measured, as for the previous ratio, in the midsagittal cut, while the middle cerebellar peduncle is assessed in a parasagittal cut and the superior cerebellar peduncle in a coronal cut. The MRI sequence used in the research validating this measurement was the T1-weighted volumetric spoiled gradient echo (Mostile et al, 2016).

The MRPI is one of the few diagnostic markers for PSP that has been shown, at least in 1 report, to accurately distinguish diagnostically equivocal or atypical cases of PSP from non-PSP. Morelli et al (2011) followed patients with "clinically uncertain parkinsonism" with a range of MRPI values. None of the 28 patients with MRPI below 13.55 later developed PSP by standard clinical criteria, and 11 of the 14 with MRPI above 13.55 did satisfy PSP diagnostic criteria after follow-up of 2 to 5 years.

The MRPI also distinguishes PSP from vascular parkinsonism. In the seminal study, MRPI greater than 13 had 100% sensitivity and specificity in this comparison. The ability of the MRPI to distinguish PSP-P from PD is less than for PSP-RS, however, presumably because of the lesser brainstem involvement in PSP-P (Longoni et al, 2011).

Use of the MRPI in clinical practice has several obstacles. One is that the literature above is based on patients with PSP-RS, and the ability of MRPI to differentiate other PSP phenotypes from their own diagnostic alternatives is unproven. More important is that achieving the coronal and parasagittal imaging planes described by Morelli et al (2011) is technically difficult and not a routine part of clinical MRI procedures. Moreover, the thin diameter of the superior cerebellar peduncle may render it difficult to measure reliably. Nor have the results of Morelli et al (2011) been validated, even in a separate, smaller validation cohort by the authors after using a larger cohort to generate the model. Another is that while the accuracy of the MRPI in distinguishing PSP from non-PSP is an improvement relative to the midbrain/pons ratio or clinical evaluation, it may be no better than a combination of the two. For these reasons, using the MRPI to diagnose PSP remains a research tool.

Providing a major step forward is a 2017 report from Mangesius et al that devised a 2-step algorithm to distinguish PSP from MSA and PD using measurements on T1-weighted images. They compared multiple candidate measures, concluding that the best results in distinguishing PSP from the other conditions came from only the midbrain and pontine diameters. The diagnostic accuracy was high even for their subjects whose scan was performed at an early stage where the diagnosis was equivocal based on clinical criteria alone and who were then followed until a diagnosis declared itself clinically. The first step in the algorithm was to exclude as PSP any patients whose ratio of pontine/midbrain diameters was less than 1.98 (nearly equivalent to the midbrain/pontine diameter ratio of 0.52 cited in other studies but calculated inversely). Then, they excluded patients whose absolute midbrain diameter was at least 9.00 mm. Of the remaining 49 patients, 45 proved to have PSP, for a positive predictive value of 92%. Of the 253 patients excluded at the first or second step, only 10 proved to have PSP, for a negative predictive value of 96%. The sensitivity can be calculated as 45 / (45 + 10), or 82%, and the specificity as 253 / (4 + 253), or 98%. While these figures are nominally similar to those of the available clinical criteria, they were based on a series that included early, equivocal cases and phenotypically atypical cases, while clinical criteria and most previous radiographic series used only patients with established PSP-RS. Another virtue of the series of Mangesius et al (2017) is that it was quite large, with 55 subjects with PSP, 194 with PD, and 63 with MSA. A drawback is that only those 2 alternative diagnoses were represented in the validation procedure (Figure 16.8).

For now, I use this new algorithm, which is easy to compute and apply, but temper my conclusions using clinical criteria and counsel patients that better diagnostic tests are on the way.

MRI: PARENCHYMAL CHANGES

Signal changes in brain tissue may also assist in the differential diagnosis of PSP. Iron deposition in the ventrolateral putamen on T2* ("T2-star") and susceptibility-weighted imaging increases strikingly in MSA-P but not in PSP (or PD). However, in the thalamus, substantia nigra, globus pallidus, caudate, and red nucleus, iron deposition is high in PSP. In PD, that signal is closer to normal in the globus pallidus and caudate, and in MSA, it is closer to normal in the other nuclei listed.

High T2 signal caused by gliosis tends to occur in moderate and advanced cases of all forms of MSA in the belly of the pons, creating the "hot cross bun sign," and at the lateral margin of the putamen, creating the "putaminal rim." These do not occur in PSP.

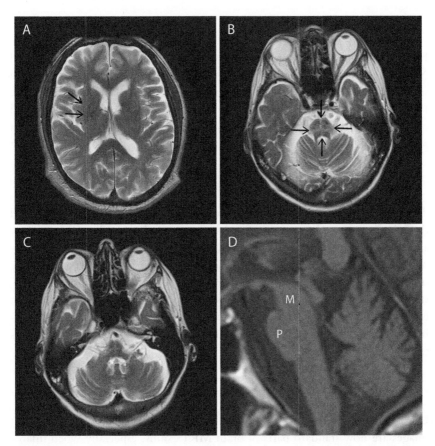

FIGURE 16.8 These show MRI features of multiple system atrophy, which can be confused with PSP because the two share postural instability, rigidity, bradykinesia, saccadic abnormalities, bladder/bowel abnormalities, rapid progression and levodopa resistance. These four MRI features occur in MSA but not in PSP: A: The "putaminal rim," a thin hyperintense line of gliosis along the lateral putamen bilaterally, more marked on the patient's right. B: The "hot cross bun sign" in the upper pons, caused by a gliotic reaction to neuronal loss. C: The same in the lower pons. The hot cross bun sign is not quite specific for MSA, as it may also occur in other rapidly progressive cerebellar degenerations. It is important to note that the phenotype of MSA most likely to be confused with PSP is MSA-parkinsonism, which is less likely to produce these changes than MSA-cerebellar. D: Atrophy that is severe in the pons (P) and mild in the midbrain (M) in a patient with MSA.

MRI: SPECTROSCOPY

Hydrogen magnetic resonance spectroscopy (H^1-MRS) shows reduced N-acetylaspartate (NAA) signal in the putamen and globus pallidus in PSP. The same has been found in PD with dementia and in MSA (Firbank et al, 2002). However, the diagnostic utility of this technique in differentiating equivocal cases of PSP from its mimics is far from established, and H^1-MRS remains a research tool.

MRI: MAGNETIZATION TRANSFER IMAGING

This newer technique images the difference between protons in free water and those bound to myelin or other fixed structures and is in effect a measure of axon density. That ratio, termed the *magnetization transfer ratio* (MTR), is abnormal in multiple areas in PD and in the atypical parkinsonisms. It is much lower in the substantia nigra in PSP than in PD or MSA, allowing complete separation of PSP from the other 2 disorders and from controls in 1 study (Eckert et al, 2004). However, the study used only 10 patients with PSP and the finding has not been replicated. Still, the dramatic results to date suggest that this technique has promise.

MRI: DIFFUSION IMAGING

Diffusion-weighted imaging (DWI) and apparent diffusion coefficient (ADC) images are now standard parts of brain MRI exams, especially when infarction is the issue. In PSP, ADC is elevated in the midbrain, globus pallidus, caudate, and superior cerebellar peduncle (SCP), findings not present to that extent in PD or MSA. The SCP signal in particular has been reported to fully separate PSP from MSA, at least by 3.0-Tesla MRI (Tsukamoto et al, 2012; Paviour et al, 2007). The utility of the more commonly available 1.5-Tesla imaging is uncertain in this regard. Still, when ordering an MRI as part of a workup for PSP or other parkinsonism, it is important to specify that DWI and ADC sequences should be included, as radiologists often omit these when stroke is not part of the stated differential.

Diffusion tensor imaging (DTI) uses ADC data, supplementing it with data to show any structural interruptions with color coding to indicate direction ("fractional anisotropy") and velocity ("mean diffusivity") of flow. DTI is routinely used in planning neurosurgical approaches, where axons serving an important function such as speech may be displaced by a tumor from their usual position in an otherwise unpredictable direction. As expected, DTI correlates well with neuronal loss in the degenerative disorders but may be a more sensitive technique for small structures. DTI in the middle cerebellar peduncles, cerebellum, and pons separates PSP from MSA moderately well, but the utility of the technique in separating PSP from other conditions is not well established. Furthermore, there is still no evidence that any abnormality would be useful before clinical signs appear or indeed before diagnosis by current clinical criteria is possible. Nor do DTI abnormalities appear to progress with the clinical disease state, even in PD, where the separation from controls is well established (Cochrane and Ebmeier, 2013). DTI, then, belongs on our long list of promising future diagnostic techniques for early or equivocal PSP that require more investigation.

METABOLIC IMAGING BY POSITRON EMISSION TOMOGRAPHY

[^{18}F]-fluorodeoxyglucose uptake as imaged by positron emission tomography (FDG-PET) reflects a combination of blood flow and glucose utilization. Most of the latter arises from synaptic activity. In PSP-RS, these images show reduced signal in frontal lobes, all of the basal ganglia, thalamus, and midbrain. Of these anatomic areas, the most consistently observed, but not the most specific, is the thalamic involvement. The frontal areas most intensely involved are premotor, precentral, prefrontal, and anterior cingulate areas. In corticobasal degeneration, a condition sometimes clinically indistinguishable from PSP, the areas of frontal hypometabolism are similar, but CBD in most cases shows marked asymmetry and involvement of parietal lobes. In MSA-P, another common PSP mimic, the putamina and pontocerebellar system show more loss than in PSP. FDG-PET may assist in differentiating PSP from PD with dementia or from Alzheimer disease (AD). Both of those latter conditions show much less frontal hypometabolism than PSP, instead featuring temporal and parietal loss. The striatum displays normal FDG-PET activity in both PD and AD but suffers major loss in PSP.

In autosomal-dominant PSP, where asymptomatic, at-risk subjects can be identified, FDG-PET changes can occur before clinical symptoms. This provides encouragement that FDG-PET may be useful as a screening tool in trials of neuroprotective agents, if only we could identify a small population of sporadic PSP to screen with this expensive technique.

The frontal and midbrain defects on FDG-PET in PSP-RS are frequently absent in other PSP phenotypes. For example, in PSP-P, the frontal loss is minimal, and in PSP–postural instability/gait freezing, the midbrain loss is present in only 25% of patients. FDG-PET pictures are less consistent or less well supported by data in the remaining minority phenotypes. The ratio of signal intensity in the putamen and thalamus has been proposed as a way to differentiate PSP-RS from PSP-P, with the first showing less putaminal activity and more thalamic activity than the latter.

Analysis of functional brain networks using FDG-PET is being developed as a differential diagnostic tool for PSP. This technique identifies a cluster of hypometabolic anatomic areas showing covariance specific to each parkinsonian syndrome. This is analogous to a specific set of quantitative abnormalities on a peripheral blood count serving to diagnose hematologic disorders. For PSP, that set comprises hypometabolism in the medial prefrontal cortex, frontal eye fields, ventrolateral prefrontal cortex, caudates, medial thalamus, and the upper brainstem. One study performed FDG-PET in diagnostically equivocal patients where PSP was on the differential diagnosis. After an average of 2.6 years' follow-up, by which time a diagnosis had declared itself by clinical criteria, the functional network analysis at baseline proved to be 88% sensitive and 94% specific for PSP (Tang et al, 2010).

DOPAMINERGIC RADIOTRACER IMAGING

One older technique labels dopaminergic postsynaptic receptors in the caudate and putamen (ie, the striatum) using PET. The ligand most commonly used is ^{11}C-raclopride. However, those neurons and receptors are not lost in early and middle stages of PD. In PSP, they are involved in the disease process, although not necessarily at a sufficiently early disease stage to be useful in the differential diagnosis of equivocal cases. For that reason, postsynaptic dopaminergic imaging is rarely used and not reimbursed as a clinical diagnostic tool.

Presynaptic dopaminergic imaging is more useful, although its clinical application is still too narrow to be of much use in PSP. The older technique uses PET to image the uptake of ^{18}F-fluoroDOPA by presynaptic terminals in the caudate and putamen. A major issue is the half-life of [18]F.

The newer technique uses single photon emission computed tomography (SPECT) to image uptake of a radio-iodine compound, ^{123}I-β-CIT or ^{123}I-FP-CIT. This technique, called a dopamine transporter (DaT) scan, provides less spatial resolution than ^{18}F-DOPA PET, but the radiochemical practicalities are far easier. DaT imaging cannot distinguish among the degenerative parkinsonian disorders but readily differentiates them all from essential tremor. It also separates dementia with Lewy bodies from AD. It may also be useful in separating parkinsonism caused by degenerative processes (including PSP) from parkinsonism caused by vascular lesions, normal-pressure hydrocephalus, neuroleptic drugs, and psychogenic causes, but these indications are not as well supported and are not reimbursed. False positives can arise from concomitant use of drugs that block dopamine reuptake such as most antidepressants and amphetaminergics and some sympathomimetic decongestants and anticholinergics, including amantadine. Withholding those drugs for a few days to weeks before the scan, as specified by the ligand manufacturer, probably avoids those interactions, although the duration specified for each drug is based on pharmacokinetic data rather than on direct clinical experience using DaT scans. Most hospitals and large radiology practices offer DaT imaging, but unfortunately, not all offer adequate levels of skill in imaging technique or interpretation. An automated interpretation technique coming online in some centers may ameliorate some of the latter difficulty.

TAU IMAGING USING PET

Compounds with an affinity for the tau protein can be radiolabeled and used as PET ligands. Perhaps the most promising to date in PSP is ^{18}F-AV-1451 or T-807, with the brand name Flortaucipir F-18, produced by Avid Radiopharmaceuticals (Schonhaut et al, 2017). However, the compound was developed for use in AD, in which the molecular characteristics of the aggregated tau differ from those of PSP. Perhaps as a result, the ligand is not as specific for the tau of PSP, with neuromelanin the most prominent target other than tau itself. Nevertheless, Passamonti et al (2017) have shown that after analysis by a sophisticated statistical technique called a "support vector machine," the anatomic pattern of ^{18}F-AV-1451 uptake in PSP could be distinguished readily from that of AD but less so from healthy controls. The study did not attempt to distinguish PSP from its competing considerations such as MSA, PD, and corticobasal degeneration, the last being a tauopathy. Nor did this or any study show longitudinal progression of the ligand uptake over the course of the illness.

Another tau PET ligand, developed in Japan by scientists at the Tohoku University, is ^{18}F-THK5351 (Brendel et al, 2018; Ishiki et al, 2017). It also is promising as an AD ligand but again is less than fully specific for tau, binding to monoamine oxidase B and perhaps to other molecules. It separated PSP from healthy controls by its midbrain signal. The midbrain uptake correlated with the PSP Rating Scale score in their 11 patients with $R = 0.66$ ($P = .026$). There was no attempt to perform serial scans or to distinguish PSP from other parkinsonian disorders.

Tau PET remains, then, in the early stages of development with regard to PSP, but it is a promising technique that clinicians should be aware of, and even before it is approved for commercial, clinical use, it may be used as an enrollment criterion for small PSP treatment trials.

CARDIAC SYMPATHETIC IMAGING

The noradrenergic sympathetic innervation of the heart as measured by ^{123}I-meta-iodobenzylguanidine (MIBG) myocardial scintigraphy is consistently reduced in PD and dementia with Lewy bodies, even without orthostatic hypotension, at least from the moderate stages or later. The abnormality is almost never present in MSA despite its prominent, consistent dysautonomia, presumably because the autonomic lesion is in the hypothalamus and brainstem rather than in the peripheral systems. In PSP, where dysautonomia other than that affecting bladder and bowel is a relatively minor issue, 6 of 7 patients in a meta-analysis nevertheless gave an abnormal result (Nagayama et al, 2005). MIBG scintigraphy, then, may help distinguish PSP from MSA, although a direct comparison has not been published and the procedure is not a standard part of clinical workups even in referral centers.

Genetics 17

For now, this remains just beyond the point of relevance to the clinical care of patients with progressive supranuclear palsy (PSP), although knowledge in this area is expanding rapidly. But as patients, and more particularly their children, often ask about the heritability of PSP, a little discussion is relevant here.

MENDELIAN FAMILIES

Documented cases of 2 or more members of a family with typical, autopsy-confirmed PSP are rare, with only about a dozen such reports in the literature (Tetrud et al, 1996; Tacik et al, 2016). There has been only 1 report, from Spain, of extended kindred with a Mendelian segregation pattern and full penetrance (Ros et al, 2005). Its causative gene has been located at chromosome 1q31.1, but in the 12 years since, the specific gene has not been published.

Rare families have an autosomal-dominant tauopathy resembling PSP except for young onset and a picture that more closely resembles frontotemporal dementia than PSP. Prominent and early features are apathy, disinhibition, hyperorality, or hypersexuality. Some have axial dystonia, rigidity, and bradykinesia not responding to levodopa. Few have gaze palsy. Their mutations are all in the MAPT gene, which encodes the tau protein. In normal adult human tau, about half of the finished molecules have 4 sites that bind to microtubules, the "microtubule-binding repeats." But in sporadic PSP, despite an absence of MAPT mutations, nearly all of the tau molecules in neurofibrillary tangles have 4 microtubule-binding repeats. The mutations in the families with MAPT mutations cluster around exon 10, which encodes 1 of the 4 repeats. The result in these monogenic cases is that exon 10 fails to be spliced out of the finished protein. PSP is therefore classed as a "4-repeat tauopathy." The cause of the phenomenon in sporadic PSP remains unknown.

FAMILIAL TENDENCIES IN SPORADIC PSP

A subtle tendency to familial clustering of sporadic PSP has been reported in case-control risk factor surveys, none reaching statistical significance. However, 1 survey (Donker Kaat et al, 2009) of 172 patients with PSP found that 7% had a close relative with PSP (although the same question was not asked of controls) and that the likelihood of subjects having a first-degree relative with dementia or parkinsonism was 33% for those with PSP and 25% for controls, giving a statistically significant odds ratio of 1.5. Considering first-degree relatives with parkinsonism (with or without dementia), the odds ratio rose to 3.9. Another evaluation (Baker et al, 2001) of 23 asymptomatic first-degree relatives of patients with PSP using tests of reaction time, olfaction, and mood found abnormal results in 39% of the patients' relatives and in none of the 23 age-matched controls. So there appears to be at least a risk of neurodegenerative signs, if not overt disease, among relatives of patients with PSP. The likelihood of patients' relatives developing PSP itself remains unknown but is sufficiently low that I tell my patients' children not to allow that risk to change their career or financial plans.

MOLECULAR GENETICS IN THE CLINIC

Genetic sequencing of the MAPT gene is commercially available, but in patients with onset of PSP after age 50 years and no affected close relatives, it is not helpful. Likewise, although a PSP pathological phenotype was described as 1 of the first 4 autopsied cases of parkinsonism associated with the LRRK2 G2019S mutation, LRRK2 mutations were not found in subsequent series of PSP, and it is not advisable to test for mutations in patients with sporadic PSP.

THE MAPT H1 HAPLOTYPE

In sporadic PSP, the first important genetic association was reported in 1999 (Baker et al, 1999). It is a haplotype (a fixed series of variants on the same chromosome) in the MAPT gene that consists of a segment that is inverted (reversed on the chromosome), with some parts duplicated. As it turns out, this "variant," dubbed H1, is actually present in the majority of the population, occurring on 77% of chromosomes in populations of European descent. But in PSP, it is present on 94% of all chromosomes. A slightly lower percentage applies in corticobasal degeneration (CBD). So the H1 haplotype appears to be (nearly) necessary to cause PSP and CBD but far from sufficient. In fact, in populations of Asian and African descent, 100% of chromosomes carry H1, yet the disease does not appear to be more common there than in European-derived populations (Evans, 2004). H1 has also been reported to increase the risk of Parkinson disease, Alzheimer disease with no ApoE-4 alleles, and even essential tremor. The molecular role of the H1 haplotype in the pathogenesis of PSP and the other conditions is not certain, but it appears to increase the transcription of tau, particularly 4-repeat tau, which is more likely to aggregate than the 3-repeat isoform (Myers et al, 2007).

OTHER GENES

A study seeking association of PSP with any of 531,451 single-nucleotide polymorphism (SNP) markers was published in 2011 (Hoglinger et al, 2011). It used DNA from 2165 cases with PSP, most of which had been proven by autopsy, and 6807 healthy, living controls. It confirmed the H1 association and found a second locus in MAPT not previously suspected and not statistically associated with the H1 haplotype. It also found highly statistically significant associations with 3 other genes: STX6, which is involved in protein handling; EIF2AK3, involved in the unfolded protein response; and MOBP, a component of myelin. The role of these in the pathogenesis of PSP remains unclear, although all 3 are plausible contributors to the current hypothesis of PSP causation. More recently, the accrual of more autopsy-proven cases allowed a reanalysis with greater statistical power. It revealed two additional genes, SLCO1A2, involved in anion transport, and DUSP10, involved in tau trafficking (Sanchez-Contreras et al, 2018).

With advances in technology, a whole-exome sequencing project in PSP has been performed. Like the SNP study, it used DNA from autopsy-proven cases. Results are expected in 2018. Also under way is a whole-genome sequencing study to examine the 99% of the genome in the untranslated, presumably regulatory areas (the introns) as well as the 1% in the coding regions (the exons). Results may arrive in 2019 or 2020.

EPIGENETICS

Epigenetic abnormalities are starting to come under scrutiny as contributors to the cause of PSP (Li et al, 2014). Attachment of small molecules, especially methyl groups, to genomic DNA alters gene expression (ie, the amount of protein encoded and/or the specific combination of exons translated into protein). Early indications are that the MAPT gene is differentially methylated in PSP, but other abnormalities are sure to be reported over the coming years. Epigenetic changes are typically caused by environmental influences, including toxins and metabolic stress, and are inherited along with the nucleotide sequences to which they attach and whose function they modify.

Drug Treatment for Motor Features 18

LEVODOPA

Levodopa treatment of Parkinson disease (PD) was one of the major medical advances of the 20th century. In PD, the striatal neurons, bearing the postsynaptic dopamine receptors, remain intact, but in progressive supranuclear palsy (PSP), they degenerate. The same is true for other neurons of the basal ganglia circuits. This probably explains why PSP responds only modestly to levodopa and loses that benefit quickly, typically by the third or fourth year of illness. PSP-parkinsonism variant may retain levodopa response a bit longer.

There has never been a double-blind trial of levodopa in PSP, but retrospective, uncontrolled record reviews typically show that about 40% of patients with PSP respond at least slightly and transiently. The placebo response rate in PSP has been reported to be as high as 30% in the older literature, but a 2016 observation using the PSP Rating Scale and the Schwab-England Activity of Daily Living Scale found no placebo response at all (Stamelou et al, 2016).

PSP symptoms that may respond to levodopa are limb rigidity and bradykinesia. Informal experience suggests that the levodopa dosage required in PSP is typically twice that in PD for the severity of abnormality. Other, usually more important, PSP symptoms such as postural instability, dysphagia, frontal dementia, and gaze palsy do not generally respond to levodopa (Lamb et al, 2016).

Although levodopa is given with carbidopa, a peripherally acting inhibitor of DOPA decarboxylase, nausea and/or vomiting remain the most common adverse effects of levodopa, occurring in about 10% of patients with PD and PSP. Fortunately, the central motor side effects of therapeutic levodopa dosages, although occurring in a majority of patients with PD after 5 years of disease, are very rare in PSP at any stage. The most common such effect in PD is chorea, most commonly at the neck and shoulders, but dystonia, myoclonus, and even tics may occur. The most likely reason for this disparity is the loss in PSP of much of the basal ganglia circuitry mediating such movement. The opposite is true of levodopa-induced hallucinations and delusions, which seem as common in PSP as in PD, although formal data are lacking.

In a retrospective chart review of 82 patients with PSP treated with carbidopa/levodopa at my center in the 1980s and early 1990s (Nieforth and Golbe, 1993), we found that benefit was mild in 31%, moderate in 7%, and marked in none, while adverse effects were mild in 17%, moderate in 6%, and marked in none. The mean maximum daily dosage of levodopa (with carbidopa) was 1015 mg. A review of published trials in 1993 (Litvan and Chase, 1993) showed a similar result, with some degree of benefit in 42%. Only rigidity and gait improved and the duration of benefit was typically 1 year, rarely 2 years. In a chart review of 11 patients receiving levodopa/carbidopa for autopsy-proven PSP (Kompoliti et al, 1998), improvement was marked in 1 and modest in the other 3. One of the latter actually showed benefit to early vertical gaze palsy that lasted 3 months.

The dosage of carbidopa/levodopa typically used in PSP starts with the 25/100 formulation at 1 tablet twice daily. It is taken on a full stomach after breakfast and supper to minimize nausea by allowing dietary large neutral amino acids to compete with levodopa, also a large neutral amino acid, slowing its transport into the brain. It should be titrated to efficacy, toxicity, or 4 tablets three times daily. If a dosage level provides no benefit after a week, it should be reduced to the highest dosage that did provide a benefit relative to the previous level and maintained there under observation for at least 2 months. If 12 tablets per day give no benefit, the dosage can be tapered by 2 tablets per day every week to the point of discontinuation 6 weeks later.

Unlike in PD, where levodopa typically provides a dramatic benefit, it may be difficult for the patient with PSP and caregivers to discern an improvement subjectively. It is impractical (although not impossible) to have the patient return to the clinic for a careful exam every week during the titration period. Therefore, the clinician must rely on a phone conversation or email with patient and caregiver. The validity of these modes of follow-up for PSP has not been assessed. There may be great potential for telemedicine in this setting.

It must be emphasized here that in PSP, levodopa would help only the rigidity and bradykinesia, which are not present to a great degree in the majority of patients. The drug could help whatever component of the gait difficulty is attributable to rigidity and bradykinesia but would not reduce postural instability as an independent deficit.

Levodopa may produce dystonia as an adverse effect in PSP that may occasionally be mistaken for features of the disease itself. The most common examples are probably laryngeal dystonia, rotational torticollis, and blepharospasm. Patients with PSP who develop those features after starting levodopa may benefit from an empirical tapering of the drug.

Although the incidence of levodopa-induced dyskinesias in patients with PSP is lower than in PD, especially considering the higher dosages used, that drug's other side effects are no different from what occurs in PD. Although dysautonomia is rare and mild in PSP except for constipation and bladder dysfunction, orthostatic hypotension frequently occurs during levodopa treatment. This is a special concern in a disease with severe postural instability.

AMANTADINE

Amantadine has multiple neuropharmacologic actions, including blockade of acetylcholinergic and N-methyl-D-aspartate (NMDA) glutamatergic receptors, promotion of dopamine release, and blockade of presynaptic dopamine reuptake. It is far from clear which of these, if any, explains its modest benefit in PSP. Amantadine has a nonspecific activating effect in some neurological conditions, and one cannot rule out the possibility that its observed effect in PSP is a similar phenomenon.

As is the case for levodopa, there has not been a controlled trial of amantadine in PSP. My own unpublished retrospective data show benefit that was mild in 9%, moderate in 31%, and marked in 7%, with adverse effects mild in 2%, moderate in 56%, and marked in 2%. For me and many other PSP specialists, this warrants a trial of amantadine in any patient with PSP who appears willing and able to tolerate the likeliest peripheral anticholinergic adverse effects, dry mouth, and constipation. The occurrence of any degree of amantadine's central anticholinergic effects, including confusion and psychosis, would justify prompt discontinuation of the drug, but their possibility would not contraindicate a cautious trial in most patients.

Amantadine is typically started at 100 mg/d, increasing if tolerated after 2 weeks to 1 capsule twice a day. If that gives no benefit after 2 more weeks, return to 100 mg/d for a week and discontinue the drug. Patients who receive benefit at 200 mg/d with tolerable side effects can be tried on 100 mg TID. At more than 100 mg/d or with evening dosing, sleep disturbances become a risk. With chronic use, tibial edema and livedo reticularis are frequent. Patients who respond to amantadine should be informed of the risk of these effects in advance lest they embark on a complicated workup for cardiac, venous, lymphatic, or renal causes of edema. Impulse control difficulty is a rare complication of amantadine where, like the edema, a relationship to that drug may not be recognized by the patient or physician.

A virtue of amantadine is that while the large size of the tablets and capsules may present difficulties for patients with PSP, the drug is also available as a syrup at 50 mg per 5 mL.

COENZYME Q-10

A defect in mitochondrial energy metabolism has been known to exist in PSP since the 1980s. It centers on complex I of the electron transport chain, where coenzyme Q-10 is a cofactor, shuttling electrons from complex I and complex II to complex III in the inner mitochondrial membrane. Treatment of rats or cultured neurons with a complex I inhibitor induces pathologic changes in the phosphorylation and location of tau from axon to cytoplasm, where it tends to form aggregates (Höglinger et al, 2003). It also depletes adenosine triphosphate (ATP), which allows accumulation of reactive oxygen species, in turn damaging structural proteins and mitochondrial membranes, feeding a vicious cycle.

A 2008 double-blind trial (Stamelou et al, 2008) found that after 6 weeks' treatment, the liposomal form of coenzyme Q-10 at 5 mg/kg/d improved the PSP Rating Scale by 1.6 points relative to placebo ($P = .008$), a difference equivalent to 4% of the baseline value. On the Frontal Assessment Battery, the benefit was similar, 6% of baseline ($P = .04$). As a demonstration that the energy production target was engaged, the patients underwent magnetic resonance spectroscopy, which showed significant improvements in the ratio of phosphocreatine to total creatine ($P < .002$) and in the ratio of ATP to adenosine diphosphate ($P < .001$). Both are markers of mitochondrial energy metabolism.

Another double-blind trial of coenzyme Q-10 gave encouraging results but a high dropout rate reduced the statistical power of the study, producing a nonsignificant outcome (Apetauerova et al, 2016).

I routinely offer my patients with PSP liposomal coenzyme Q-10 at 100 mg TID. This form is claimed to cross the blood-brain barrier, while the standard form used in cardiology does not. It is available only in liquid form and is sold without a prescription. Its monthly cost of approximately $80 is a sacrifice for some patients, so it is important to assess the result after 2 months and to discontinue treatment if there has been no benefit.

DRUGS COMMONLY RECOMMENDED IN THE PAST

Amytriptyline, a tricyclic antidepressant, has multiple central actions. It has been promoted for PSP on the strength of a 1985 double-blind study that enrolled only 4 patients in a crossover design (Newman et al, 1985). The strength of the recommendation seems to be based more on the study's rare virtue as a controlled trial, however small, while almost all of the other literature on approved drugs in PSP are chart reviews or small case series. Amitriptyline 50 mg HS provided "definite" improvement relative to placebo in 2 patients and "probable" improvement in 1 patient. As in a more recent study (Stamelou, 2016), there was no placebo effect relative to baseline. In my own center's 78 patients receiving amitriptyline for PSP, benefit occurred in about one-third and adverse effects in over half, typically moderate in severity. One of the 4 patients in Newman et al (1985) suffered significant worsening of postural instability. This adverse effect has occurred with sufficient frequency in my hands, sometimes with resulting falls and injury, that I no longer use amitriptyline in PSP. Confusion, somnolence, and agitation are other common adverse effects of amitriptyline seen in PSP, where such issues are already part of the patient's daily challenge.

Zolpidem, a GABA agonist commonly prescribed as a sleep aid, has been tried against PSP, where there is loss of GABA-ergic neurons in the striatum and globus pallidus. The original report, from Daniele et al (1999), was a 10-patient, double-blind crossover study. Only 2 patients showed a clinically meaningful improvement in the Unified Parkinson's Disease Rating Scale (UPDRS) motor score, but the mean improvement relative to baseline was 6.5% for the 5-mg group and, oddly, only 0.8% for the 10-mg group. Adverse effects, especially somnolence and an increase in postural instability, were common. After this publication, I tried zolpidem up to 10 mg/d in 20 patients with PSP, finding moderate benefit in 30% and marked benefit in 5%. However, adverse effects were moderate in 75% and marked in 5%. I no longer use zolpidem routinely in PSP other than as a sleep aid.

Dopamine receptor agonists have shown no greater likelihood of efficacy in PSP than levodopa, with more adverse effects (Jankovic, 1983; Weiner et al, 1999). Their greater risk, relative to levodopa, for psychosis, orthostatic hypotension, somnolence, and impulse dyscontrol, makes them a poor option for patients with PSP. Nevertheless, many neurologists are in the habit of initiating treatment of parkinsonian disorders with an agonist or substituting an agonist when levodopa treatment is giving poor results. I therefore often find myself having to taper and discontinue a dopamine agonist in a newly referred patient with PSP. The result is usually an improvement in alertness.

Methysergide, a serotonergic, gave positive results in PSP in a double-blind trial published in 1981 (Rafal and Grimm, 1981). Especially exciting was an apparent benefit to the downgaze palsy in at least 1 patient. The drug enjoyed a number of years of enthusiasm, with a reported response rate in nonblinded experience of about 25%. But the original trial's blinding methodology was shown to be faulty, and the drug's benefits on informal experience seemed to disappear. The drug has dropped off the list of routine empirical treatments in PSP.

DEEP BRAIN STIMULATION

Despite the dramatic efficacy of deep brain stimulation (DBS) in Parkinson disease, this approach has proven inefficacious in PSP and the other "atypical" parkinsonisms. The presumptive reason is that the basal ganglia outflow nuclei, which are overactive in PD and the sites used for DBS in that condition, are part of the primary pathologic picture in PSP. They therefore are already underactive and the inhibitory effect of DBS would only make matters worse. However, in recent years there is interest in DBS in the pedunculopontine nucleus (PPN) in PSP. Dysfunction of that nucleus is related to balance and multiple other brainstem functions. Preliminary results in small numbers of patients are only weakly encouraging, with little morbidity, modest measurable benefit and no improvement in patients' daily activities (Galazky et al, 2018).

CONCLUSIONS

My routine for drug treatment of PSP, as yet to be formally evaluated, starts one drug at a time and evaluates its effect, at least by phone, before starting another. The first is carbidopa/levodopa titrated to efficacy, toxicity, or 1200 mg (with carbidopa) per day in those cases where rigidity and bradykinesia contribute importantly to the patient's difficulties in daily activities. If that is not the case, I start with amantadine 100 mg/d. If this is tolerated, I increase to 100 mg BID after 2 weeks and have the patient call 2 weeks later to report. If there has been no benefit, I reduce it to 100 mg/d for 3 days and then discontinue it. If the patient has been on amantadine for longer, I taper more slowly to avoid the withdrawal effect that is common with that drug. If the patient does report benefit from amantadine, I continue it and do not attempt to increase it further, as that usually causes more adverse effects than additional benefit in this population.

At that point, with or without amantadine, I add coenzyme Q-10, liposomal form, 100 mg TID and ask the patient or caregiver to report back by phone in 2 months or to do that at the next visit. If there is no subjective benefit, I discontinue the coenzyme Q-10 and ask for a phone call if any abrupt deterioration occurs. In that case, I will resume the coenzyme Q-10. A problem in titrating the coenzyme Q-10 is that the onset of benefit is gradual and may

TABLE 18.1 Algorithm for empirical symptomatic drug treatment of general and motor features of PSP

The indicated order is recommended.

1. Carbidopa/levodopa
   a. Does the patient's rigidity or bradykinesia importantly affect the daily activities?
      i. Yes
         1. Start carbidopa/levodopa 25/100 one BID on full stomach.
         2. Titrate to efficacy, toxicity, or 4 tablets TID.
         3. After reaching 2 tablets BID, can switch to the 25/250 tablets, 1 BID and titrate to 5 tablets per day divided into 3 doses.
            a. If benefit has occurred, add amantadine.
         4. If no benefit, taper by 200 to 250 per day each week.
            a. If symptoms worsen, increase by 1 dose level and maintain.
            b. A week after carb/levo is discontinued, consider starting amantadine.
      ii. No: Go to amantadine.

2. Amantadine
   a. Does the patient have moderate or severe dementia or severe constipation despite best management?
      i. Yes
         1. Go to coenzyme Q-10.
      ii. No
         1. Start amantadine 100 mg once daily.
         2. After 2 weeks, if no important adverse effects, increase to 100 mg BID.
         3. Reevaluate, at least by phone, in 2 weeks.
            a. If patient has benefited with few side effects, increase to 100 mg TID.
            b. If no benefit, reduce to 100 mg daily for 2 weeks, then discontinue.
            c. If there is benefit but with dry mouth or constipation, attempt to treat those.
            d. If cognitive adverse effects occur, taper and discontinue drug.

3. Coenzyme Q-10
   a. Use the liposomal form (a liquid, 100 mg per 5 mL or 1 mL), 100 mg TID.
   b. Reevaluate in 6 weeks. If no benefit, discontinue.

require several weeks. Over that span of time, the natural history of the disease and its typical minor symptomatic exacerbations and recoveries will obscure any symptomatic benefit of the coenzyme Q-10. This is why trials of discontinuation of the supplement should be implemented periodically, perhaps once a year, to continually reassess the benefit of this $80 per month expenditure.

Further detail on a recommended protocol for empirical drug treatment of the motor features of PSP appears in Table 18.1.

In assessing the response to drug manipulation, repeating the PSP Rating Scale at each visit appears to be more valuable than relying on subjective reports, but outcome data are not available. In evaluating the symptomatic effects of treatment, the clinician must correct for the natural history of PSP, which produces an approximately 1-point progression on the PSP Rating Scale each month.

Management of Nonmotor Features 19

As in Parkinson disease (PD), the rigidity, bradykinesia, tremor, and postural instability (ie, the "parkinsonian" features) form only a minority of the problems facing patients. The same is true in progressive supranuclear palsy (PSP), but the nonmotor features are different from those in PD. Whereas nonmotor issues in early and moderate PD center on autonomic and visceral function, they emphasize cognitive and behavioral function in PSP. In the later stages, when cognitive and behavioral issues become more important in PD, in PSP the issues tend to move to the brainstem, with disturbances in sleep, swallowing, speech, and, of course, eye movement (Lang, 2005).

DEMENTIA

The profound loss of acetylcholinergic neuronal systems in PSP prompted enthusiasm in the 1980s and 1990s for the then newly marketed cholinesterase inhibitors as treatment for the dementia or motor features of PSP (Huey et al, 2006). But careful trials (Fabbrini et al, 2001; Litvan et al, 1989) have given largely negative results, and these drugs are no longer generally recommended in PSP. However, hope may remain for those with frontotemporal dementia as part of their PSP phenotype, where an open study of rivastigmine showed improvement in some behavioral measures, resulting in lesser caregiver burden but not in measures of cognition. Some PSP experts try an anticholinesterase in those few patients with PSP whose cognitive state emphasizes memory or spatial deficits, by analogy with Alzheimer disease.

Memantine, a glutamate antagonist related to amantadine that is approved for the dementia of Alzheimer disease, has also been tried for the dementia of PSP without success. In my patients with PSP, it almost uniformly has caused nausea, dizziness, and somnolence with no benefit. However, 1 open trial from Boxer et al (2009) showed that memantine at 20 mg daily gave modest benefit to some cognitive and behavioral measures in progressive nonfluent aphasia (PNFA) as part of the tau-based form of frontotemporal lobar degeneration. A trial of memantine in patients with PNFA as part of PSP now seems warranted.

DEPRESSION

Depression has been little studied in PSP. One controlled cross-sectional survey (Bloise et al, 2014) found that of 28 patients with PSP, depression was present in 15, and in 8 of these, it was attributed to the PSP disease process itself. Only 5 of the 28 age-matched controls were found to have depression ($P=.005$). Neither monoamine oxidase inhibitors, tricyclics, selective serotonin reuptake inhibitors, nor serotonin-norepinephrine reuptake inhibitors have been systematically studied for the depression of PSP. The few reports of these drugs in PSP focused on motor features rather than depression (Miyaoka et al, 2002). Nevertheless, most specialists do attempt treatment for depression in PSP with these drugs as for depression in PD. Our retrospective data show a relatively good risk/benefit ratio for fluoxetine. Bupropion has also anecdotally been reported to be of value.

AGITATION AND PSYCHOSIS

Nocturnal hyperactivation is common with PSP. No controlled data are available, but experience suggests melatonin up to 12 mg at bedtime as the first line, followed by zolpidem to 10 mg HS and then by a tricyclic such as imipramine hydrochloride 25 mg HS. If these fail, a benzodiazepine such as temazepam 15 to 30 mg HS can be used nightly for periods of up to 2 weeks or, if used only occasionally, for indefinite periods. If insomnia is related to agitation or psychosis, quetiapine starting at a quarter of a 25-mg tablet HS may be used for short periods. It can be titrated up to 100 mg HS, proceeding to a half tablet, then 1 tablet, then increasing in increments of 1 tablet to efficacy or toxicity. Risk of death from a variety of causes has been reported for the demented, elderly patients treated with antipsychotics. In the setting of PSP, this small risk is not an absolute contraindication, but dosages should be kept low and other approaches should be tried first (Bloise et al, 2014).

For the elderly, the most frequent adverse effects of quetiapine are daytime somnolence, orthostatic hypotension, and electrocardiogram abnormalities. Personal experience suggests that quetiapine exacerbates motor parkinsonism in 5% to 10% of patients with PSP. Clozapine is the antidopaminergic that joins quetiapine as the only antidopaminergic antipsychotics with an acceptably low risk of exacerbating the motor parkinsonism in patients with such preexisting disorders. However, clozapine has not been formally evaluated in PSP. Its requirement for weekly white blood cell testing for the first 6 months (less often thereafter) and its risk of sudden death in the elderly render it impractical. Other antipsychotics, including those that are "atypical" for their low risk of tardive dyskinesia, have an unacceptably high risk of exacerbating motor parkinsonism in patients with PSP and should be avoided. The value of pimavanserin for medication-related psychosis in PSP has not been determined, although it is approved for that indication in PD.

SIALORRHEA

Some patients with PSP list drooling as their worst daily torment. Treatment starts with advice to suck on a lollipop or other hard candy. While this may increase salivary flow and is often prescribed as treatment for dry mouth, it also stimulates the patient to swallow. A pharmacologic approach is an anticholinergic with predominantly peripheral action such as glycopyrrolate starting at 1 mg 3 times a day (TID), with oxybutynin 5 mg twice a day (BID) to TID. Both drugs can be taken as needed. Both carry the risk of adverse effects via other peripheral anticholinergic effects such as constipation and mydriasis causing blurred vision. Both also carry a slight risk of passing the blood-brain barrier enough to cause confusion, lethargy, or psychosis. A treatment often recommended is atropine eye drops given sublingually as a way to inhibit salivary activity by local action. In my experience in patients with PSP, this causes systemic peripheral and central toxicity too often to justify its efficacy.

Intraparotid botulinum toxin was effective in an open series of 6 patients with PSP (Gómez–Caravaca et al, 2015). The initial dosage in each parotid was 14.5 units of Botox, with a mean of 22.2 units eventually found to be required. Ultrasound guidance was not used. The average duration of benefit was 4.4 months.

DRY EYES

In PSP, the markedly reduced blink rate deprives the conjunctival surface of access to the oils and waxes from the Meibomian glands and from the glands of Zeis and Moll. These secretions are spread by blinking and, as a group, reduce evaporation of the tear film and performance of other functions to maintain the conjunctival surface. Reduced efficiency of this process causes not only a dry eye sensation but also conjunctivitis, with resulting painful photophobia. Some patients with PSP may not close the lids completely during sleep because of their supranuclear lid control deficit. The process can be exacerbated by anticholinergic medication, which reduces tear secretion. In such cases, an initial measure is to attempt to discontinue any such drugs such as amantadine or those for the urinary urgency or sialorrhea of PSP.

Typical initial treatment is frequent use of normal saline drops, which only mimic the aqueous lacrimal gland secretion for less than an hour or over-the-counter lubricants containing various cellulose solutions, acetylcysteine, or carbomer gel, which mimic the oily secretions and may last longer.

If those measures fail, referral to an ophthalmologist or optometrist is warranted. Such specialists may prescribe a hydroxymethyl cellulose gel tablet (eg, Lacrisert) to be inserted by the patient or caregiver into the lower conjunctival sac; insert puncta plugs, which reduce drainage of both the aqueous and oily tears from the conjunctival sac; provide a contact bandage made from amniotic sac material (eg, Prokera) that dissolves slowly while allowing the dried, inflamed cornea to heal; or prescribe cyclosporine (eg, Restasis) drops, which may reduce inflammation caused by drying. No published literature supports any of these in patients specifically with PSP. Data on the efficacy of surgical approaches for dry eyes in PSP are similarly lacking, but a common procedure is a tarsorrhaphy to narrow the palpebral fissure and allow the lids to close completely during sleep.

EYE MOVEMENT ABNORMALITIES

For diplopia, a monocular prism can allow the patient to fuse the images resulting from asymmetric eye movement restriction. However, the gaze palsy of PSP is difficult to treat. Binocular prisms are frequently prescribed in an attempt to raise the lower half of the patient's space to a point within range of their gaze. This helps for only a few days, as the patient's central compensatory mechanisms return the perception of the scene to its original position.

Bifocals and progressive lenses are difficult for those with PSP for the obvious reason of poor downgaze, but a pair of glasses for near tasks can help during eating or reading, making the proper focus available in the position of primary gaze. The analogous but opposite solution may help the patient with the retrocollis of PSP who needs distance refraction during walking.

Some of the visual loss of PSP may result from the combination of small deficits, not one of which alone would be noticed. For example, a loss of contrast sensitivity that interferes with feeding can be addressed by yellow eyeglass filters, dark plates for light-colored foods and light plates for dark-colored foods, and 2 kitchen cutting boards, 1 dark and 1 light, to improve the patient's ability to see various foods while cutting. Contrasting tape can be placed on the lips of stairs and on other edges around the home.

The patient and family should also be informed of the multiple services for the vision impaired such as audio books at public libraries, audio descriptions of the visual scene offered by some video-streaming services, and an audio news feed app available from the National Federation for the Blind (https://nfb.org/nfbnewsline).

URINARY INCONTINENCE

Disrupted bladder physiology in PSP varies widely in type and severity, but urinary retention and bladder overfilling are rare (Wakatsuki et al, 1993). Urgency and incontinence are treated as for any other neurogenic disorder with a few caveats. Peripherally acting anticholinergics are the mainstay of drug treatment here, but in patients with diffuse cerebral degenerative disorders, they can at times display central effects such as confusion, agitation, and psychosis. Anticholinesterases for dementia such as donepezil, rivastigmine, and galantamine can cause urinary urgency and help the dementia of PSP little if at all. As in anyone with urinary urgency, diuretics such as antihypertensives, caffeine, and alcohol should be minimized. Trips to the bathroom during the night can be dangerous for those with PSP, given the postural instability, impulsivity, downgaze problems, and, in many cases, unavailability of the still-sleeping caregiver. Therefore, the clinician should maintain a low threshold for prescribing such measures such as fluid restriction after suppertime and nocturnal use of desmopressin 0.1 mg (nasal spray and intramuscular preparations are also available) (Batla et al, 2016). Early evaluation by a neurourologist can reveal unrelated, more treatable urinary tract issues. Injection of botulinum toxin injections of the detrusor has been found helpful in the incontinence of PD but has not been formally evaluated in PSP.

CONSTIPATION

This very common part of PSP is treated as for any other elderly patients with only a few caveats. The program starts with adequate hydration, which may be difficult to achieve in PSP because of the patient's dysphagia for liquids and desire to reduce urinary urgency. Another important measure is to enforce adequate physical activity, also a challenge in a patient with poor balance. A high-fiber diet or fiber supplement is also useful and easier to implement. When dietary control fails, a bulk-forming agent, typically a form of plant fiber, can be taken daily and chronically. Popular preparations are psyllium, inulin, wheat dextrin, methylcellulose, and polycarbophil.

The next step is a gentle stool softener such as docusate (dioctyl sulfosuccinate). It starts at 100 mg daily, titrating at weekly intervals to BID and then TID. Each dose must be taken with at least half a glass of water. Patients should be warned that the effect usually requires a few days to appear and to continue dosing even on days with a satisfactory bowel movement. Docusate can be used chronically, as it has no biological activity on the bowel, acting only osmotically. The docusate capsules may be too large for some patients with PSP to swallow safely, but docusate is also available as a liquid and as an enema. The most commonly available form is docusate sodium, which contains 5 g of sodium for each 100-mg gel capsule. Alternatives for patients who cannot tolerate sodium are calcium and potassium salts of docusate.

Another popular osmotic stool softener is a polymer, polyethylene glycol (Di Palma et al, 2002). It is sold as a powder to be mixed in water or juice. The usual dosage is 17 g once daily, and the label warns against usage for more than 2 weeks. Like docusate, it must be used daily for 3 or 4 days in most patients before a result appears. However, a double-blind trial showed that a dose of 68 g produces the first bowel movement in an average of 14 hours and the second in 19 hours. All patients reported complete relief by the second movement and no adverse effects. Whether these results can be extended to patients with PSP or other neurodegenerative diseases remains a question.

Other osmotically acting constipation remedies are aqueous solutions of salts of citrate, magnesium, sulfate, or phosphate. They can act rapidly, typically in 30 minutes to 3 hours, and can cause dehydration and electrolyte disturbances. Lactulose is a slower-acting hyperosmotic and, unlike the salts, can be used daily, but its latency to benefit may be 2 days. These all require a large volume of water as a solvent.

If these fail or if the volume of oral solution required cannot be tolerated by a patient with the dysphagia of PSP, a bowel stimulant may be tried on a short-term basis. They typically require 6 to 10 hours to work and can result in refractory colonic paresis with chronic use. Popular stimulants include senna and bisacodyl. Another is castor oil, but in patients with aspiration risk, oils by mouth are not recommended, even in small volumes, for fear of causing lipoid pneumonia.

An alternative to stimulant laxatives is an enema using saline or a hyperosmolar salt solution. Multiple kits are sold over the counter. Many patients find that the esthetic downside is justified by the prompt and complete results.

Emergency Management 20

This chapter is designed for clinicians caring for a patient with an established diagnosis of progressive supranuclear palsy (PSP) who presents with an urgent neurological complaint. It is designed as a quick reference for acute-care medical professionals who are unfamiliar with the disorder.

BACKGROUND

PSP is a rare brain degeneration with a prevalence in the United States of only 4000 to 5000 persons, compared with 600,000 for Parkinson disease (PD). Often called one of the "atypical parkinsonisms" or "Parkinson-plus" disorders, PSP may resemble PD in its general slowing, rigidity, and balance issues. PSP starts at an average age of 63 years and encounters life-threatening complications of immobility and dysphagia an average of 7 years later. The dementia and behavioral changes that complicate PSP often produce a misdiagnosis of Alzheimer disease or depression. The principal neurological features cluster into those arising from brainstem degeneration (dysarthria, dysphagia, eye movement problems, sleep problems), basal ganglia (sudden falls, rigidity, bradykinesia, occasionally tremor), and frontal cortex (impulsivity, loss of "executive" cognition with memory and language relatively spared). It responds little or not at all to anti-PD medications, but most patients receive 1 or more such drugs anyway as a trial.

COMMON FEATURES

Falls

The most common and, for most patients, the initial feature of PSP is a loss of balance with falls. As a result, trauma is the most common reason for emergency care through most of the disease course. The falls are disproportionately backward. Even after the patient is wheelchair bound, the motor impulsivity of PSP causes many patients to attempt to walk imprudently.

The other motor features of PSP are more parkinsonian and not cerebellar in appearance, but the gait of PSP can appear cerebellar, like that of alcohol intoxication. There is also a rare variant that features difficulty with initiation of gait, or freezing of gait on encountering turns or thresholds.

Further increasing the risk of falls is the difficulty moving the eyes, particularly downward. The difficulty in maintaining ocular fixation reduces visual perception, contributing to fall risk. The impulsiveness and loss of judgment exacerbate the effects.

Vertigo

PSP only rarely causes true vestibular dysfunction, but the poor balance together with the difficulty of ocular fixation is often described as "dizziness." However, this complaint is almost always chronic in PSP. An acute onset of such symptoms deserves a more detailed workup.

Dementia

PSP features a "frontal" dementia, with loss of inhibition and difficulty organizing complex cognitive tasks. Depression and agitation are frequent signs. Bradyphrenia, where the patient's responses are appropriate but delayed, sometimes by several minutes, is also common and can give the appearance of dementia, aphasia, depression, or somnolence. This may interfere with the evaluation of the patient in an emergency setting.

Dysphagia/Aspiration

Aspiration pneumonia is the most common cause of death in PSP, and aspiration without pneumonia is another complication of PSP requiring emergency care. Like most neurological causes of dysphagia, liquids present more difficulty than solids. The aspiration pneumonia of PSP is treated like that of any cause. However, PSP reduces cough efficiency, requiring more attention by the staff to suctioning of secretions than is often the case for patients with intact brainstem reflexes.

Dysarthria

The dysarthria of PSP may resemble that of PD, with soft volume and rapid pace, but more commonly it also has a spastic (explosive or elastic-sounding) and/or ataxic (drunken-sounding) quality. Advanced patients are often completely mute but can understand well. Like bradyphrenia, dysarthria can interfere with evaluation of a patient in the emergency room.

Rigidity

In PSP, rigidity of the neck is often disproportionate and can produce a suspicion of meningitis, especially in a patient with confusion of unclear duration. However, the muscle rigidity of PSP is not associated with fever, nausea, Kernig or Brudzinski signs or funduscopic evidence of increased intracranial pressure.

Rigidity of trunk and limbs makes provision of care difficult and can be the factor that induces the family to bring a patient to the ER in the hopes of nursing home placement. In such patients, inquiry regarding recent drug discontinuation or noncompliance may be fruitful.

As for any chronic, diffuse, disabling brain disorders, neurological exacerbations in PSP can result from unrelated stresses such as urinary tract infection (UTI), pneumonia, dehydration, constipation, or pain, as from decubiti or arthralgias.

Visual Symptoms

Difficulty in moving the eyes can bring a patient to the ER with a complaint of visual loss or diplopia, although the problem is never truly acute. Physical findings include restriction of up- and downgaze, jerky pursuit, poor convergence, and square-wave jerks, which are very rapid horizontal binocular movements of 5 degrees or less. Nystagmus can also occur and eye movement problems can be moderately asymmetric. PSP does not affect the refractive apparatus, iris, retina, or optic nerve. If there is disconjugate gaze, referral can be made electively to an ophthalmologist or optometrist for consideration of prisms, but these would not help the difficulty with conjugate gaze.

Although PSP can affect eye movement asymmetrically, it would not cause unequal pupils or pupils that are not round.

Intermittent or constant blepharospasm or inhibition of lid elevation is common in PSP and can cause functional blindness. There is no acute treatment except for reassurance and perhaps mild sedation, but chronic, repeated injections of botulinum toxin into the muscles of the eyelids can be performed by an ophthalmologist. Like any botulinum treatment, this would not take effect until after several days.

The blink rate in PSP is severely reduced, often to 20% of normal. This can cause drying with pain, itching, reactive conjunctivitis, lacrimation, and photophobia. The last symptom, especially together with cognitive slowing and nuchal rigidity, can mimic meningitis or subarachnoid hemorrhage.

Bladder Dysfunction

PSP causes upper motor neuron–type bladder dysfunction, with urgency and, later, urge incontinence. If a distended bladder is detected, an unrelated spinal cord problem or outflow obstruction should be suspected. UTIs are very common in PSP and urosepsis joins falls and aspiration pneumonia as the major causes of morbidity and mortality in PSP.

The anticholinergic drugs, including amantadine, are commonly used in PSP and may cause retention. The MAO-B inhibitors, which are not useful in PSP but are sometimes prescribed anyway by analogy with PD, can also cause retention.

The dysphagia and aspiration risk of PSP causes many patients and their caregivers to limit fluid intake, exacerbating UTI risk. This should be discouraged, and perhaps the best person to do that is the ER doctor treating the patient for a painful UTI. Such patients should be referred for a dysphagia evaluation. Reluctance to undertake a trip to the bathroom during the night also prompts patients with PSP to limit fluid intake. This should be addressed via a physical therapy evaluation.

Constipation

PSP causes constipation via involvement of parasympathetic centers in the lower spinal cord. It can cause impaction that may bring the patient to the ER and is treated like constipation of any cause. Consideration should be given to reducing or discontinuing any anticholinergics in use. Dehydration caused by fear of aspiration also contributes to constipation in PSP.

Pain

PSP does not cause neurogenic pain. However, pain can arise from severe constipation with impaction and from constant dystonic contraction of the muscles of the neck or occasionally of the hands, wrists, and ankles. Other secondary causes of pain in PSP include UTIs, trauma from falls, and decubiti.

TOXICITY OF DRUGS USED FOR PSP

Antiemetics

Rigidity and bradykinesia, as the hypodopaminergic features of PSP, can be exacerbated dramatically by any drug blocking dopamine receptors. Antiemetics such as metoclopramide (Reglan) and prochlorperazine (Compazine) are 2 frequent offenders. For nausea or vomiting, use trimethobenzamide (Tigan), ondansetron (Zofran), or granisetron (Kytril). When muscle rigidity is suddenly increased by dopamine receptor blockade, the dysphagia and aspiration risk can be aggravated dramatically. There is also a risk of increased muscular rigidity causing rhabdomyolysis and malignant hyperthermia.

Tranquilizers

Most of the neuroleptic tranquilizers should be avoided for the same reason as the antidopaminergic antiemetics. Some frequent offenders are haloperidol (Haldol), olanzapine (Zyprexa), aripiprazole (Abilify), and risperidone (Risperdal). Two neuroleptics, quetiapine (Seroquel) and clozapine (Clozaril), have only a low risk of exacerbating the rigidity and bradykinesia of the parkinsonian disorders and can be used in PSP. For agitation in PSP, benzodiazepines provide the best risk/benefit ratio despite their sedation risk in the elderly.

Anticholinergics

The most common are amantadine (Symmetrel), trihexyphenidyl (Artane), and benztropine (Cogentin). They can cause confusion, myoclonus, lethargy, hallucinations, or agitation, as in any patients who are elderly or have existing diffuse disorders of the cerebral cortex. Anticholinergics are frequently prescribed for the motor features of PSP, although the only one recommended here is amantadine.

One other word about amantadine is that its abrupt discontinuation can cause a withdrawal effect comprising worsening of the motor features of PSP, including dysphagia with resulting aspiration risk. If a patient with PSP presents with toxicity suspected of resulting from amantadine, the dosage should be reduced by no more than half immediately, with instructions to follow up with the neurologist or primary care physician by phone a week later for consideration of further tapering or discontinuation of the drug.

For patients with PSP, the most commonly used nonpsychiatric drugs with anticholinergic properties are those inhibiting bladder emptying such as tolterodine (Detrol), oxybutynin (Ditropan), solifenacin (Vesicare), and darifenacin (Enablex). The alpha-sympathetic blockers used for urinary incontinence such as alfuzosin (Uroxatral), doxazosin (Cardura), and guanfacine (Tenex) are not offenders on that score but can cause hypotension.

A scopolamine skin patch is sometimes prescribed for the "vertigo" (actually, postural instability) of PSP. It is not effective in that indication, but it can of course cause anticholinergic adverse effects. As a transdermal patch, it may not be recalled by the stressed patient or caregiver when listing medications and may not be apparent to the examiner, as it is usually hidden behind the ear.

Dopaminergics

The dopaminergic drugs used for the parkinsonisms such as carbidopa/levodopa (Sinemet), pramipexole (Mirapex), ropinirole (ReQuip), rasagiline (Azilect), and selegiline (Eldepryl) can cause hallucinations, hypotension, sedation, and confusion. Frequently in PD but only rarely in PSP, they can also cause choreatic involuntary movements. These most commonly occur in the muscles of the neck and shoulder girdle but can also occur in the lower extremities, face, and even diaphragm, producing a complaint of dyspnea.

Dopaminergic Withdrawal

Patients with PSP are often treated with dopaminergic or anticholinergic antiparkinson medication. Although the response in PSP is modest and short-lived, the abrupt discontinuation of these drugs can produce an acute reaction similar to neuroleptic malignant syndrome. This may include severe rigidity, with fever, delirium, tremor, dysphagia with aspiration risk, autonomic instability, and rhabdomyolysis with myoglobinuric renal damage. Therefore, a patient suspected of having dopaminergic toxicity should have the offending drug reduced acutely by no more than a third.

The same reaction can result in a patient with any degenerative parkinsonian condition whose remaining dopaminergic synaptic function is blocked by neuroleptic tranquilizers and antiemetics such as metoclopramide and prochlorperazine.

Amantadine

This drug also has nonanticholinergic properties that can cause toxicity. Pedal edema, which can extend well above the knees, is a common effect of longterm amantadine use. It is nonpitting, nonpainful, and not associated with the usual medical causes of edema. It resolves over a period of weeks after discontinuation of the drug. Another is livedo reticularis, a lacy-appearing skin discoloration most common in the legs. It is harmless and, like the edema, will resolve a few weeks after discontinuing the drug.

Some neurological signs and symptoms common in the elderly *not* caused by PSP appear in Table 20.1.

TABLE 20.1 Some acute neurological signs/symptoms common in the elderly not caused by PSP

Sign/symptom	Likely causes in the setting of PSP
Aphasia, acute	A rare form of PSP features primary progressive aphasia, but its onset is gradual and progressive.
Chorea	However, high-dosage dopaminergic drugs can cause chorea in PSP, although less frequently than in Parkinson disease.
Focal weakness, chronic Focal muscle atrophy Fasciculations	These can occur in amyotrophic lateral sclerosis, which can otherwise mimic PSP in its gait problem, dysphagia, and, in some cases, frontal dementia. Frontotemporal dementia, which can resemble PSP in its cognitive deficits, has a variant with prominent motor neuron disease.
Focal deficits, transient	Apraxia, occurring in a significant minority with PSP, is usually asymmetric. Its resulting motor impairment can appear intermittent, as they are a function of the task presented. This can superficially resemble a transient cerebrovascular event.
Hearing loss or tinnitus	PSP can cause apathy and poor gaze fixation, which can mimic a hearing deficit.
Hypesthesia or paresthesia	The immobility of PSP can cause root or nerve compression.
Limb ataxia	A rare variant of PSP features cerebellar deficits, but otherwise, the only cerebellar features in PSP are the square-wave jerks and some elements of speech and gait. The finger-nose test may be degraded in PSP by difficulty in binocular convergence on a near target.
Migraine-type headache	However, occipital headache may result from constant hyperextension of the neck.
Visual complaints, monocular	However, visual fixation instability can produce the complaint of "blurring" or monocular diplopia.
Myoclonus	When occurring in the setting of apparent PSP, a metabolic problem, postanoxic state, or medication toxicity is most likely, but consider the alternative diagnoses of multiple-system atrophy and corticobasal degeneration.
Pain, chest	Consider aspiration pneumonia or pulmonary embolus resulting from the immobile state.
Pain, abdomen	Consider fecal impaction or urinary tract infection.
Pain, back	Consider urinary tract infection, pulmonary embolism, or exacerbation of lumbar spondylosis by the immobile state.
Seizures or syncope	The apathy, gaze palsy, and disordered sleep in PSP may conspire to mimic a partial complex seizure.
Seizures or syncope	Dementia with Lewy bodies (DLB) can mimic PSP in some ways. One of DLB's cardinal features is episodes of impairment of consciousness or delirium lasting minutes to hours without hemodynamic compromise or electroencephalographic changes.

RADIOLOGIC FINDINGS OF PSP

Brain magnetic resonance imaging (MRI) in moderate and advanced stages of PSP causes diffuse cerebral atrophy and disproportionate atrophy of the midbrain and anterior temporal lobes and dilation of the posterior third ventricle. It can also cause increased iron deposition in the putamen symmetrically. Sometimes there is evidence of gliosis (high T2 signal) in the basal ganglia. Ventricular enlargement is proportionate to cortical atrophy. The computed tomography scan only reveals the atrophy mentioned above. A multi-infarct state can mimic PSP clinically but would not cause the focal areas of atrophy.

PSP causes no abnormalities of the bony spine except for retroflexion at the neck in some cases.

Organization and Infrastructure of Care 21

THE ROLE OF THE MOVEMENT DISORDER SUBSPECIALIST

Like any patients with a chronic neurological condition, those with progressive supranuclear palsy (PSP) can encounter an array of complications for which the neurologist should act as a "modified primary care physician." The absence, so far, of a specific treatment for PSP makes this role even more critical.

Internal medicine subspecialists often act as the true primary care physician for patients whom they first encountered in the context of a subspecialty problem such as a myocardial infarction. That's part of the culture of internal medicine but not typically of neurology and PSP need not be an exception. Although it is not customary or appropriate for the neurologist to continue as the primary physician, a movement disorder specialist who diagnoses PSP in a patient without another neurologist should offer to act as the patient's general neurologist for the duration. This is because knowledge of what PSP does and does not do is critical to the diagnostic evaluation of such patients. For example, the neurologist should know that sudden onset of pain or highly asymmetric motor loss would not be caused by PSP and should be worked up as in anyone else. Conversely, patients with established PSP complaining of dizziness, falls, or urinary incontinence can be spared most or all of the workup.

One hopes that every primary care practitioner with at least 1 patient with PSP will become sufficiently knowledgeable on the disorder (perhaps by reading this book) as not to need a neurologist at the ready for such situations. In reality, this is unlikely to occur, and the neurologist must fill that gap. This arrangement requires a good working relationship with the primary care physician. It also requires the *existence* of a primary care physician. Many patients, even in their 50s or 60s, when PSP typically begins, will have no primary care physician whom they trust for complicated issues. Neurologists must insist that their patients with PSP acquire a primary physician if they do not already have one and be prepared to make that referral.

OTHER SPECIALISTS

The neurologist's file folder with the list of trusted primary care physicians should include another of medical and surgical specialists. Patients with PSP frequently require referral to specialists in infectious disease, geriatric psychiatry, orthopedic surgery, ophthalmology, and urology. The last 2 specialties have subspecialties in neuro-ophthalmology and neurourology, which are often more useful than the "general" specialists in the PSP population. However, these subspecialists are rare outside of major metropolitan areas or academic clinics.

The neurologist must also maintain a network of other allied professionals conversant with PSP and willing to accept such patients. Perhaps most useful is a speech/swallowing pathologist who can evaluate and help manage dysphagia, the most common cause of serious morbidity and mortality in PSP. Physical therapy is another important resource. Both are more readily available than neurologists, so patients who travel a distance to see the neurologist typically prefer to stay closer to home for their swallowing evaluations and physical therapy. This makes it difficult for the neurologist to ensure that the quality of the service is adequate for patients with rare conditions. CurePSP's website (www.curepsp.org) offers quick guides to PSP for such allied professionals, as does this book.

It is also advisable to offer patients with PSP access to a geriatric social worker to assist with issues of insurance, employment, assistive devices, psychological support, end-of-life decisions, and hospice care.

PHYSICAL FACILITIES OF A PSP REFERRAL CENTER

The standard modern outpatient suite needs no modification for the care of patients with PSP. The PSP Rating Scale requires no equipment other than a cup of water to assess dysphagia. An examining table is necessary to check supine blood pressure as part of ruling out the diagnosis of multiple-system atrophy or dementia with Lewy bodies, both common mimics of PSP.

If one were designing or choosing an outpatient facility for patients with PSP or other severe motor disorders, its corridors would be wide enough for 2 wheelchairs to pass. There would be a corridor or other space at least 20 feet long where a patient's gait can be videoed without risk of collisions with hurried staff. Exam rooms would be large enough to video a sitting patient without cutting off head or feet. Adequate light would be available to achieve good video resolution of details such as eye movement. There would be a separate room for an assistant to administer neuropsychological tests without distractions from family or phone. There would also be a meeting room where multiple professionals, a wheelchair-bound patient, and accompanying caregivers and family can confer.

Perhaps surprisingly, it may not be advisable to install handrails along the walls of the same corridor used for testing gait. Many patients with PSP would grasp the rails purely as a result of frontal motor disinhibition, creating a false impression of postural instability. Testing the gait of a patient with true postural instability should be assisted by an aide who has been instructed not to allow contact unless necessary to prevent a fall.

The goal is to allow patients with difficulty traveling or difficulty arranging transportation to receive all of their PSP-related care in 1 location. Few centers are organized to offer the ideal, where patients see multiple specialists and allied health services on the same visit. However, most centers can realistically, and with administrative cooperation, provide an on-site physical therapy facility where initial evaluations are offered. There should also be easy access to speech/language pathology, neurourology, neuro-ophthalmology, and behavioral neurology or geriatric psychiatry.

COMMUNITY EDUCATION AND SUPPORT GROUPS

The ideal PSP referral center should include a program devoted to wellness comprising at least a lay-organized support group. Professionals associated with the center should be available as guest speakers. Experience shows, however, that caregivers of those with PSP are too committed to that task to take on the additional burden of coordinating a support group. Furthermore, with PSP as rare as it is, the number of patients willing and able to travel to a central location is rarely sufficient to provide "critical mass" for a support group.

One solution may be to design support groups for caregivers rather than for patients themselves. Caregivers can travel to meetings more easily and need psychological support and technical information at least as much as patients. CurePSP maintains a network of support groups around the United States and Canada and provides resources for those willing to take on the task of creating new groups. Many academic centers and large hospitals maintain an office of community outreach that may be able to provide coordination, meeting facilities, and nominal expenses for a PSP support group.

As professionals looking after people with as rare a condition as PSP, part of our responsibility is to encourage patients' family members to lead support groups despite the time demands of caregiving. Support and coordination for support groups are available from CurePSP, headquartered in New York City; The PSP Association in London, England; and PSP Canada in Kingston, Ontario. Similar organizations are starting to form in other countries as well.

THE POTENTIAL ROLE OF TELEMEDICINE

Telemedicine offers a promising option for care of patients who find travel difficult and have disorders familiar to only a few subspecialist clinicians at distant centers. PSP is therefore an ideal candidate for this despite the potential difficulties of assessing eye movements by video and managing the risk of falls during the exam. As of this writing, telemedicine has not yet been implemented specifically for PSP professional care or lay support. However, this will certainly change as the generation comfortable with technology reaches the PSP age group and as the technology improves in its efficiency and ease of use.

"CurePSP CENTERS OF CARE"

An initiative by CurePSP in the United States announced in late 2017 is to identify tertiary centers offering excellent care for PSP. Although the initial goal is guidance for patients in finding care, subsequent goals of the CurePSP Centers of Care program will be standardization and validation of care protocols and pooling of clinical research efforts. Criteria for designation, none mandatory by itself, include staff experience in PSP, size of the PSP patient clientele, availability of expertise such as behavioral neurology and ancillary services, clinical research experience in PSP, availability of the center to trainees, a record of published research in PSP, and geographical distance from existing CurePSP Centers of Care. As of September 2018, 16 centers had been approved.

What's Coming? 22

This short book has been specifically designed as a guide for the practicing clinician rather than as a scientific treatise. There is little on molecular biology, pathology, or genetics. The few forays into that territory have been carefully chosen to assist clinicians in answering patients' educated questions. The few discussions of experimental treatment merely supplement the accompanying discussion of existing options, so a second edition will soon be in order. As a bridging maneuver, here are my personal favorites for the next important steps in the clinical care of people with progressive supranuclear palsy (PSP).

First, diagnosis. Over the next few years, positron emission tomography (PET) using tau tracers, disappointing to date except in distinguishing groups of diagnostically established patients, will probably become sufficiently refined to differentiate PSP from the synucleinopathies (Schonhaut et al, 2017; Brendel et al, 2018). This will be assisted by the parallel development of alpha-synuclein PET tracers. Distinguishing PSP from tauopathies such as frontotemporal dementia and Alzheimer disease will become feasible if only via their different anatomic distribution, but ruling out corticobasal degeneration (CBD) with a Richardson syndrome phenotype will be more difficult. All this may require newer tau tracers, as the ones presently under evaluation may not be sufficiently specific for tau. The newer tracers could be designed for specificity for the "strains" of tau most prevalent in PSP, a very hot topic in "tauology" at the moment.

Radiologic diagnosis of PSP using non-PET modalities in general is in its own state of flux (Whitwell et al, 2017). New magnetic resonance imaging (MRI) modalities using diffusion tensor imaging and new ways of measuring structures using old MRI modalities are perhaps the most promising and do not require new hardware. The most promising replacement for the PSP Rating Scale in assessing benefits of experimental neuroprotective treatment is serial morphometry using conventional, although carefully standardized, T1 MRI.

Another promising area is in prognosis. For unclear reasons, cerebrospinal fluid (CSF) concentration of phosphorylated tau tends to be lower than in controls and much lower than in Alzheimer disease and frontotemporal dementia, and the lower the level, the more rapid the subsequent disease progression. Neurofilament light chain (NfL) is a nonspecific marker of central nervous system (CNS) damage whose level is proportionate to progression. The ratio of NfL to p-tau has recently been found to predict PSP progression well, at least over 1 year's observation (Rojas et al, 2018). The PSP Rating Scale has been known for over a decade to predict acquisition of disease milestones, and new longitudinal data are expected soon (from my group) to strengthen and supplement those 2007 findings (Golbe and Ohman-Strickland, 2007).

The epidemiology of PSP is ripening. Our thinking on the rarity of PSP was upended in 2014 by brain bank data suggesting that 5% of the population develops PSP brain pathology by the time of death. If this is the case, and if a more sensitive diagnostic test can be devised, the landscape will change for early diagnosis, clinical prevention trials, and genetic studies (Dugger et al, 2014). Another important, if anecdotal, report is the first geographic cluster of PSP, in an area of northern France heavily contaminated by industrial metals (Caparros-Lefebvre et al, 2015). This opens the tantalizing possibility that all PSPs may require a metal or metals as a necessary pathogenetic cofactor and, if that is true, points toward primary prevention.

Our notion of the clinical spectrum of PSP took a major step with the seminal 2005 report of PSP-parkinsonism as distinct from PSP–Richardson syndrome (Williams et al, 2005). Many more "minority phenotypes" have since been described, and more are sure to come. The challenge will be to determine which are mere sections of a spectrum and which are separate pathogenetic entities. The significance for clinicians is that awareness of atypical forms of PSP would improve diagnosis, spare unnecessary diagnostic testing, and allow patients to enter treatment trials, or treatment itself, earlier in the disease course.

Secondary prevention of PSP (ie, slowing of progression in diagnosed patients) is presently undergoing trials using antibodies against tau (West et al, 2017). These intravenously infused proteins do enter the CNS well enough to reduce extracellular tau in CSF and are well tolerated to date. Efficacy data will probably be available in 2019. Other pharmaceutical companies and academic groups have other antitau antibodies waiting in the wings. The next neuroprotective approach to enter clinical trials will probably be small drugs that inhibit

O-GlcNAcase. This enzyme inhibits the physiologic removal of the sugar N-acetylglucosamine from the tau molecule, which in turn reduces tau misfolding and aggregation (Wani et al, 2017). A bit further off are non-antibody approaches to reducing abnormal tau such as infusion of microRNA, which are tiny lengths of RNA that are physiologically produced to regulate gene expression.

Driving much of the recent research interest in PSP has its sharing of tau pathology with Alzheimer disease (AD), an epidemiologically and commercially much more important entity. PSP serves as a convenient "test bed" for anti-AD tau-based therapeutics. However, as more details of the tau pathology in the 2 disorders come to light, certain important differences are emerging (Gibbons et al, 2018). Those differences may make a tau-based treatment for one useless for the other. Whether these will return PSP to its former "orphan" status is perhaps the most important single potential development for us all to follow.

ACKNOWLEDGMENTS

A college professor of mine, a prolific researcher, once told me, "There are two types—those who write books and those who actually find the stuff out." Leading the long list of those who actually discovered a lot of what's in this book and then personally taught it to me are Adam Boxer, Tony Lang, Andrew Lees, Irene Litvan, Stefan Lorenzl, Günter Höglinger, Huw Morris, Maria Stamelou, and, perhaps most important, John Steele. For educating me in their specialties, I am grateful to Dennis Dickson, Jonathan and Bethany Fishbein, Fred Lepore, and Jerry Schellenberg. For its persistent confidence in me, I thank CurePSP and its leadership: Dave Kemp, Alex Klein, and Bill McFarland. For his mentorship and for first directing my research interest to PSP, I thank the late Roger Duvoisin. Most important, and for everything that really matters, I thank my wife, Devra Golbe.

REFERENCES

Aarsland D, Litvan I, Larsen JP. Neuropsychiatric symptoms of patients with progressive supranuclear palsy and Parkinson's disease. *J Neuropsychiat Clin Neurosci.* 2001;13:42–49.

Abbott SM, Videnovic A. Sleep disorders in atypical parkinsonism. *Mov Disord Clin Pract (Hoboken).* 2014;1:89–96.

Adams RD, Fisher CM, Hakim S, et al. Symptomatic occult hydrocephalus with "normal" cerebrospinal-fluid pressure—a treatable syndrome. *N Engl J Med.* 1965; 273:117–126.

Albers DS, Augood SJ, Martin DM, et al. Evidence for oxidative stress in the subthalamic nucleus in PSP. *J Neurochem.* 1999;73:881–884.

Albert ML, Feldman RG, Willin AL. The subcortical dementia of progressive supranuclear palsy. *JNNP.* 1974;37:121–130.

Aldrich MS. Sleep disturbances. In: Litvan I, Agid Y, eds. *Progressive Supranuclear Palsy: Clinical and Research Approaches.* New York, NY: Oxford University Press; 1992:169–183.

Alzheimer A. Über eine eigenartige Erkrankung der Hirnrinde. *Allg Zschr Psychiatr Psych gerichtl Med.* 1907;64:146–148.

Anderson TJ, MacAskill MR. Eye movements in patients with neurodegenerative disorders. *Nat Rev Neurol.* 2013;9:74–85.

Apetauerova D, Scala SA, Hamill RW, et al. CoQ10 in progressive supranuclear palsy: A randomized, placebo-controlled, double-blind trial. *Neurol Neuroimmunol Neuroinflamm.* 2016;3:e266. doi: 10.1212/NXI.0000000000000266

Arai H, Morikawa Y, Higuchi M, et al. Cerebrospinal fluid tau levels in neurodegenerative diseases with distinct tau-related pathology. *Biochem Biophys Res Commun.* 1997; 236:262–264.

Arena JE, Weigand SD, Whitwell JL, et al. Progressive supranuclear palsy: progression and survival. *J Neurol.* 2016;263:380–389.

Baker KB, Montgomery EB Jr. Performance on the PD test battery by relatives of patients with progressive supranuclear palsy. *Neurology.* 2001;56:25–30.

Baker M, Litvan I, Houlden H, et al. Association of an extended haplotype in the tau gene with progressive supranuclear palsy. *Hum Mol Genet.* 1999;8:711–715.

Bang J, Lobach IV, Lang AE, et al. Predicting disease progression in progressive supranuclear palsy in multicenter clinical trials. *Parkinsonism Relat Disord.* 2016;28:41–48.

Batla A, Tayim N, Pakzad M, Panicker JN. Treatment options for urogenital dysfunction in Parkinson's disease. *Curr Treat Options Neurol.* 2016;18:45.

Bensimon G, Ludolph A, Agid Y, et al; NNIPPS Study Group. Riluzole treatment, survival and diagnostic criteria in Parkinson plus disorders: the NNIPPS study. *Brain.* 2009;132 (Pt 1):156–171.

Bloise MC, Berardelli I, Roselli V, et al. Psychiatric disturbances in patients with progressive supranuclear palsy: a case-control study. *Parkinsonism Relat Disord.* 2014;9:965–968.

Boeve B, Dickson D, Duffy J, et al. Progressive nonfluent aphasia and subsequent aphasic dementia associated with atypical progressive supranuclear palsy pathology. *Eur Neurol.* 2003;49: 72–78.

Boeve BF, Lang AE, Litvan I. Corticobasal degeneration and its relationship to progressive supranuclear palsy and frontotemporal dementia. *Ann Neurol.* 2003;54(suppl 5): S15-S19.

Bower JH, Maraganore DM, McDonnell SK, et al. Incidence of PSP and multiple system atrophy in Olmsted County, Minnesota, 1976 to 1990. *Neurology.* 1997;49:1284–1288.

Boxer AL, Lang AE, Grossman M, et al.; AL-108-231 Investigators. Davunetide in patients with progressive supranuclear palsy: a randomised, double-blind, placebo-controlled phase 2/3 trial. *Lancet Neurol.* 2014;13:676–685. 2014.

Boxer AL, Lipton AM, Womack K, et al. An open-label study of memantine treatment in 3 subtypes of frontotemporal lobar degeneration. *Alzheimer Dis Assoc Disord.* 2009;23: 211–217.

Brendel M, Schönecker S, Höglinger GU, et al. [^{18}F]-THK5351 PET correlates with topology and symptom severity in progressive supranuclear palsy. *Front Aging Neurosci.* 2018 Jan 17;9:440.

Brown RG, Lacomblez L, Landwehrmeyer BG, et al; NNIPPS Study Group. Cognitive impairment in patients with multiple system atrophy and progressive supranuclear palsy. *Brain.* 2010;133:2382–2393.

Bruns M, Josephs K. Neuropsychiatry of corticobasal degeneration and progressive supranuclear palsy. *In Rev Psych.* 2013;25:197–209.

Bukki J, Nubling G, Lorenzl S. Managing advanced PSP and CBD in a palliative care unit: admission triggers and outcomes. *Am J Hosp Palliat Care.* 2014;33:477–482.

Caparros-Lefebvre D, Elbaz A; and the Caribbean Parkinsonism Study Group. Possible relation of atypical parkinsonism in the French West Indies with consumption of tropical plants: a case-control study. *Lancet.* 1999;354:281–286.

Caparros-Lefebvre D, Golbe LI, Deramecourt V, et al. A geographical cluster of progressive supranuclear palsy in northern France. *Neurology.* 2015;85:1293–1300.

Chambers CB, Lee JM, Troncoso JC, et al. Overexpression of four-repeat tau mRNA isoforms in progressive supranuclear palsy but not in Alzheimer's disease. *Ann Neurol.* 1999;46:325–332.

Champy P, Höglinger GU, Féger J, et al. Annonacin, a lipophilic inhibitor of mitochondrial complex I, induces nigral and striatal neurodegeneration in rats: possible relevance for atypical parkinsonism in Guadeloupe. *J Neurochem.* 2004;88:63–69.

Chen AL, Riley DE, King SA, et al. The disturbance of gaze in progressive supranuclear palsy: implications for pathogenesis. *Front Neurol.* 2010;1:147.

Clavaguera F, Akatsu H, Fraser G, et al. Brain homogenates from human tauopathies induce tau inclusions in mouse brain. *Proc Natl Acad Sci U S A.* 2013;110:9535–9540.

Cochrane CJ, Ebmeier KP. Diffusion tensor imaging in parkinsonian syndromes: a systematic review and meta-analysis. *Neurology.* 2013;80:857–864.

Compain C, Sacre K, Puéchal X, et al. Central nervous system involvement in Whipple disease: clinical study of 18 patients and long-term follow-up. *Medicine (Baltimore).* 2013; 92:324–330.

Conrad C, Andreadis A, Trojanowski JQ, et al. Genetic evidence for the involvement of tau in PSP. *Ann Neurol.* 1997;41:277–281.

Critchley M. Arteriosclerotic parkinsonism. *Brain.* 1929;52:23–83.

Cubo E, Stebbins GT, Golbe LI, et al. Application of the Unified Parkinson's Disease Rating Scale in progressive supranuclear palsy: factor analysis of the motor scale. *Mov Disord.* 2000;15:276–279.

Curran T, Lang AE. Parkinsonian syndromes associated with hydrocephalus: case reports, a review of the literature, and pathophysiological hypotheses. *Mov Disord.* 1994;9:508–520.

Daniele A, Moro E, Bentivoglio AR. Zolpidem in progressive supranuclear palsy. *N Engl J Med.* 1999 Aug 12;341:543–4.

de Yébenes JG, Sarasa JL, Daniel SE, et al. Description of a pedigree and review of the literature. *Brain.* 1995;118;1093–1103.

Di Fabio RP, Zampieri C, Tuite P. Gaze-shift strategies during functional activity in progressive supranuclear palsy. *Exp Brain Res.* 2007;178:351–362.

Di Palma JA, Smith JR, Cleveland M. Overnight efficacy of polyethylene glycol laxative. *Am J Gastroenterol.* 2002;97:1776–1779.

Dickson DW. Neuropathologic differentiation of progressive supranuclear palsy and corticobasal degeneration. *J Neurol.* 1999;246(suppl 2):II6–II15.

Donker Kaat L, Boon AJ, Azmani A, et al. Familial aggregation of parkinsonism in progressive supranuclear palsy. *Neurology.* 2009;73:98–105.

Donker Kaat L, Boon AJ, Kamphorst W, et al. Frontal presentation in progressive supranuclear palsy. *Neurology.* 2007;69:723–729.

Doty RL, Golbe LI, McKeown DA, et al. Olfactory testing differentiates between progressive supranuclear palsy and idiopathic Parkinson's disease. *Neurology.* 1993;43:962–965.

Dubois B, Slachevsky A, Litvan I, et al. The FAB: a Frontal Assessment Battery at bedside. *Neurology.* 2000;55:1621–1626.

Dubois B, Slachevsky A, Pillon B, et al. "Applause sign" helps to discriminate PSP from FTD and PD. *Neurology.* 2005;64:2132–2133.

Dugger BN, Hentz JG, Adler CH, et al. Clinicopathological outcomes of prospectively followed normal elderly brain bank volunteers. *J Neuropathol Exp Neurol.* 2014;73: 244–252.

Eckert T, Sailer M, Kaufmann J, et al. Differentiation of idiopathic Parkinson's disease, multiple system atrophy, progressive supranuclear palsy, and healthy controls using magnetization transfer imaging. *Neuroimage.* 2004;21:229–235.

Espay AJ, Da Prat GA, Dwivedi AK. Deconstructing normal pressure hydrocephalus: ventriculomegaly as early sign of neurodegeneration. *Ann Neurol.* 2017;82:503–513.

Evans W, Fung HC, Steele J, et al. The tau H2 haplotype is almost exclusively Caucasian in origin. *Neurosci Lett.* 2004;369:183–185.

Evidente VG, Adler CH, Sabbagh MN, et al. Neuropathological findings of PSP in the elderly without clinical PSP: possible incidental PSP? *Parkinsonism Relat Disord.* 2011; 17:365–371.

Fabbrini G, Barbanti P, Bonifati V, et al. Donepezil in the treatment of progressive supranuclear palsy. *Acta Neurol Scand.* 2001;103:123–125.

Fegg MJ, Kögler M, Abright C, et al. Meaning in life in patients with progressive supranuclear palsy. *Am J Hosp Palliat Care.* 2014;31:543–547.

Firbank MJ, Harrison RM, O'Brien JT. A comprehensive review of proton magnetic resonance spectroscopy studies in dementia and Parkinson's disease. *Dement Geriatr Cogn Disord.* 2002;14:64–76.

Frost B, Jacks RL, Diamond MI. Propagation of tau misfolding from the outside to the inside of a cell. *J Biol Chem.* 2009;284:12845–1252.

Gaig C, Graus F, Compta Y. Clinical manifestations of the anti-IgLON5 disease. *Neurology.* 2017;88:1736–1743.

Galazky I, Kaufmann J, Lorenzl S, et al. Deep brain stimulation of the pedunculopontine nucleus for treatment of gait and balance disorder in progressive supranuclear palsy: Effects of frequency modulations and clinical outcome. *Parkinsonism Relat Disord.* 2018;50:81–86.

Ghosh BC, Carpenter RH, Rowe JB. A longitudinal study of motor, oculomotor and cognitive function in progressive supranuclear palsy. *PLoS One.* 2013;8:e74486.

Gibbons GS, Banks RA, Kim B, et al. Detection of Alzheimer disease (AD)–specific tau pathology in AD and non-AD tauopathies by immunohistochemistry with novel conformation-selective tau antibodies. *J Neuropathol Exp Neurol.* 2018;77:216–228.

Glasmacher SA, Leigh PN, Saha RA. Predictors of survival in progressive supranuclear palsy and multiple system atrophy: a systematic review and meta-analysis. *J Neurol Neurosurg Psychiatry.* 2017;88:402–411.

Goetz CG, Leurgans S, Lang AE, et al. Progression of gait, speech and swallowing deficits in progressive supranuclear palsy. *Neurology.* 2003;60:917–922.

Golbe LI. Progressive supranuclear palsy. In: Tolosa E, Koller WC, Gershanik OS, eds. *Differential Diagnosis and Treatment of Movement Disorders.* Boston, MA: Butterworth-Heinemann; 1998:27–38.

Golbe LI, Davis PH, Lepore FE. Eyelid movement abnormalities in progressive supranuclear palsy. *Mov Disord.* 1989;4:297–302.

Golbe LI, Davis PH, Schoenberg BS, Duvoisin RC. Prevalence and natural history of PSP. *Neurology.* 1988;38:1031–1034.

Golbe LI, Ohman-Strickland PA. A clinical disability rating scale for progressive supranuclear palsy. *Brain.* 2007;130:1552–1565.

Golbe LI, Rubin RS, Cody RP, et al. Follow-up study of risk factors in progressive supranuclear palsy. *Neurology.* 1996;47:148–154.

Goldberg LS, Altman KW. The role of gastrostomy tube placement in advanced dementia with dysphagia: a critical review. *Clin Interv Aging.* 2014;9:1733–1739.

Gómez-Caravaca MT, Cáceres-Redondo MT, Huertas-Fernández I, et al. The use of botulinum toxin in the treatment of sialorrhea in parkinsonian disorders. *Neurol Sci.* 2015;36:275–279.

Grandas F, Esteban A. Eyelid motor abnormalities in progressive supranuclear palsy. *J Neural Transm Suppl.* 1994;42:33–41.

Hall DA, João Forjaz M, Golbe LI, et al. Scales to assess clinical features of progressive supranuclear palsy: MDS Task Force Report. *Mov Disord Clin Pract.* 2015;2: 127–134. doi10.1002/mdc3.12130.

Hansson O, Janelidze S, Hall S, et al. Blood-based NfL: a biomarker for differential diagnosis of parkinsonian disorder. *Neurology.* 2017;88:930–937.

Hauw J-J, Daniel SE, Dickson D, et al. Preliminary NINDS neuropathologic criteria for Steele-Richardson-Olszewski syndrome (PSP). *Neurology.* 1994;44,2015–2019.

Hauw J-J, Hausser-Hauw C, De Girolami U, et al. Neuropathology of sleep disorders: a review. *J Neuropathol Exp Neurol.* 2011;70:243–252.

Hewer S, Varley S, Boxer AL, et al. Minimal clinically important worsening on the Progressive Supranuclear Palsy Rating Scale. *Mov Disord.* 2016;31:1574–1577.

Höglinger GU, Féger J, Prigent A, et al. Chronic systemic complex I inhibition induces a hypokinetic multisystem degeneration in rats. *J Neurochem.* 2003;84:491–502.

Höglinger GU, Huppertz HJ, Wagenpfeil S, et al.; TAUROS MRI Investigators. Tideglusib reduces progression of brain atrophy in progressive supranuclear palsy in a randomized trial. *Mov Disord.* 2014;29:479–487.

Höglinger GU, Kassubek J, Csoti I, et al. Differentiation of atypical Parkinson syndromes. *J Neural Transm (Vienna).* 2017;124:997–1004.

Höglinger GU, Melhem NM, Dickson DW, et al. Identification of common variants influencing risk of the tauopathy progressive supranuclear palsy. *Nat Genet.* 2011;43: 699–705.

Höglinger GU, Respondek G, Stamelou M, et al., for the Movement Disorder Society–endorsed PSP Study Group. Movement Disorder Society—clinical diagnostic criteria for progressive supranuclear palsy. *Mov Disord.* 2017;332:853–864.

Huey ED, Putnam KT, Grafman J. A systematic review of neurotransmitter deficits and treatments in frontotemporal dementia. *Neurology.* 2006;66:17–22.

Intiso D, Bartolo M, Santamato A, et al. The role of the rehabilitation in subjects with progressive supranuclear palsy: a narrative review *PMR.* 2018;10:636–645.

Ishiki A, Harada R, Okamura N, et al. Tau imaging with ^{18}F-THK-5351 in progressive supranuclear palsy. *Eur J Neurol.* 2017;24:130–136.

Jabbari E, Zetterberg H, Morris HR. Tracking and predicting disease progression in progressive supranuclear palsy: CSF and blood biomarkers. *J Neurol Neurosurg Psychiatry.* 2017; 88:883–888.

Jankovic J. Controlled trial of pergolide mesylate in Parkinson's disease and progressive supranuclear palsy. *Neurology.* 1983;33:505–507.

Jecmenica-Lukic M, Petrovic IN, Pekmezovic T, et al. Clinical outcomes of two main variants of progressive supranuclear palsy and multiple system atrophy: a prospective natural history study. *J Neurol.* 2014;261:1575–1583.

Josephs KA, Katsuse O, Beccano-Kelly DA, et al. Atypical progressive supranuclear palsy with corticospinal tract degeneration. *J Neuropathol Exp Neurol.* 2006;65:396–405.

Josephs KA, Whitwell JL, Eggers SD, et al. Gray matter correlates of behavioral severity in progressive supranuclear palsy. *Mov Disord.* 2011;26:493–498.

Kanazawa M, Shimohata T, Toyoshima Y, et al. Cerebellar involvement in progressive supranuclear palsy: a clinicopathological study. *Mov Disord.* 2009;24:1312–1318.

Kanazawa M, Tada M, Onodera O, et al. Early clinical features of patients with progressive supranuclear palsy with predominant cerebellar ataxia. *Parkinsonism Relat Disord.* 2013; 19:1149–1151.

Kass-Iliyya L, Kobylecki C, McDonald KR, et al. Pain in MSA and PSP compared to PD. *Brain Behav.* 2015;5:e00320.

Kato N, Arai K, Hattori T. Study of the rostral midbrain atrophy in progressive supranuclear palsy. *J Neurol Sci.* 2003;210:57–60.

Kawashima M, Miyake M, Kusumi M, et al. Prevalence of progressive supranuclear palsy in Yonago, Japan. *Mov Disord.* 2004 Oct;19:1239–40.

Kimura D, Barnett HJ, Burkhart G. The psychological test pattern in progressive supranuclear palsy. *Neuropsychologia.* 1981;19:301–306.

Kluin KJ, Foster NL, Berent S, et al. Perceptual analysis of speech disorders in progressive supranuclear palsy. *Neurology.* 1993;43:563–566.

Koga S, Josephs KA, Ogaki K, et al. Cerebellar ataxia in progressive supranuclear palsy: an autopsy study of PSP-C. *Mov Disord.* 2016;31:653–662.

Kompoliti K, Goetz CG, Litvan I, et al. Pharmacological therapy in progressive supranuclear palsy. *Arch Neurol.* 1998;55:1099–1102.

Kraemer BC, Zhang B, Leverenz JB, et al. Neurodegeneration and defective neurotransmission in a Caenorhabditis elegans model of tauopathy. *Proc Natl Acad Sci U S A.* 2003;100: 9980–9985.

Krismer F, Pinter B, Mueller C, et al. Sniffing the diagnosis: olfactory testing in neurodegenerative parkinsonism. *Parkinsonism Relat Disord.* 2017;35:36–41.

Kuhn TS. *The Structure of Scientific Revolutions*. University of Chicago Press, 1962.

Kwok JB, Teber ET, Loy C, et al. Tau haplotypes regulate transcription and are associated with Parkinson's disease. *Ann Neurol.* 2004;55:329–334.

Lamb R, Rohrer JD, Lees AJ, et al. Progressive supranuclear palsy and corticobasal degeneration: pathophysiology and treatment options. *Curr Treat Options Neurol.* 2016;12:42.

Lang AE. Treatment of progressive supranuclear palsy and corticobasal degeneration. *Mov Disord.* 2005;20(suppl 1):S83.

Larner AJ. Did Charles Dickens describe progressive supranuclear palsy in 1857? *Mov Disord.* 2002;17:832–833.

Leclair-Visonneau L, Rouaud T, Debilly B, et al. Randomized placebo-controlled trial of sodium valproate in progressive supranuclear palsy. *Clin Neurol Neurosurg.* 2016;146:35–39.

Lewis J, McGowan E, Rockwood J, et al. Neurofibrillary tangles, amyotrophy and progressive motor disturbance in mice expressing mutant (P301L) tau protein. *Nature Genetics.* 2000;25:402–405.

Lewy FH. Paralysis agitans. 1. Pathologische Anatomie. In: Lewandowsky M, editor. *Handbuch der Neurologie, Dritter Band, Spezielle Neurologie I.* Berlin: Julius Springer; 1912. pp. 920–933.

Li Y, Chen JA, Sears RL, et al. An epigenetic signature in peripheral blood associated with the haplotype on 17q21.31, a risk factor for neurodegenerative tauopathy. *PLoS Genet.* 2014;10:e1004211.

Lindemann U, Nicolai S, Beische D, et al. Clinical and dual-tasking aspects in frequent and infrequent fallers with progressive supranuclear palsy. *Mov Disord.* 2010;25:1040–1046.

Ling H, de Silva R, Massey LA, et al. Characteristics of progressive supranuclear palsy presenting with corticobasal syndrome: a cortical variant. *Neuropathol Appl Neurobiol.* 2014;40:149–163.

Litvan I, Agid Y, Calne D, et al. Clinical research criteria for the diagnosis of progressive supranuclear palsy: Report of the NINDS-SPSP International Workshop. *Neurology.* 1996;47:1–9.

Litvan I, Chase TN. Traditional and experimental therapeutic approaches. In: Litvan I, Agid T, eds. *Progressive Supranuclear Palsy: Clinical and Research Approaches.* New York, NY: Oxford University Press; 1993:254–269.

Litvan I, Gomez C, Atack JR, et al. Physostigmine treatment of progressive supranuclear palsy. *Ann Neurol.* 1989;26:404–407.

Litvan I, Lees PS, Cunningham CR, for ENGENE-PSP. Environmental and occupational risk factors for progressive supranuclear palsy: case-control study. *Mov Disord.* 2016;31:644–652.

Litvan I, Mega MS, Cummings JL, et al. Neuropsychiatric aspects of progressive supranuclear palsy. *Neurology.* 1996;47:1184–1189.

Litvan I, Sastry N, Sonies BC. Characterizing swallowing abnormalities in progressive supranuclear palsy. *Neurology.* 1997;48:1654–1662.

Longoni G, Agosta F, Kostić VS, et al. MRI measurements of brainstem structures in patients with Richardson's syndrome, progressive supranuclear palsy-parkinsonism, and Parkinson's disease. *Mov Disord.* 2011;26:247–255.

Lopez OL, Litvan I, Catt KE, et al. Accuracy of four clinical diagnostic criteria for the diagnosis of neurodegenerative dementias. *Neurology.* 1999;53:1292–1299.

Maher ER, Lees AJ. The clinical features and natural history of the Steele-Richardson-Olszewski syndrome (progressive supranuclear palsy). *Neurology.* 1986;36:1005–1008.

Mangesius S, Hussl A, Krismer F, et al. MR planimetry in neurodegenerative parkinsonism yields high diagnostic accuracy for PSP [published online October 31, 2017]. *Parkinsonism Relat Disord.*

Massey LA, Jäger HR, Paviour DC, et al. The midbrain to pons ratio: a simple and specific MRI sign of progressive supranuclear palsy. *Neurology.* 2013;80:1856–1861.

Menza MA, Cocchiola J, Golbe LI. Psychiatric symptoms in progressive supranuclear palsy. *Psychosomatics.* 1995;36:550–554.

Miyaoka T, Seno H, Inagaki T, Horiguchi J. Fluvoxamine for the treatment of depression and parkinsonism in progressive supranuclear palsy. *Int J Psychiatry Clin Pract.* 2002; 6:45–47.

Morariu MA. Progressive supranuclear palsy and normal-pressure hydrocephalus. *Neurology.* 1979;29:1544–1546.

Morelli M, Arabia G, Novellino F, et al. MRI measurements predict PSP in unclassifiable parkinsonisms. *Neurology.* 2011;77:1042–1047.

Mostile G, Nicoletti A, Cicero CE, et al. Magnetic resonance parkinsonism index in progressive supranuclear palsy and vascular parkinsonism. *Neurol Sci.* 2016;37:591–595.

Muller J, Wenning GK, Verny M, et al. Progression of dysarthria and dysphagia in postmortem-confirmed parkinsonian disorders. *Arch Neurol.* 2001;58:259–264.

Myers AJ, Pittman AM, Zhao AS, et al. The MAPT H1c risk haplotype is associated with increased expression of tau and especially of 4 repeat containing transcripts. *Neurobiol Dis.* 2007;25:561–570.

Nagayama H, Hamamoto M, Ueda M, Nagashima J, Katayama Y. Reliability of MIBG myocardial scintigraphy in the diagnosis of Parkinson's disease. *J Neurol Neurosurg Psychiatry.* 2005;76:249–251.

Nath U, Ben-Shlomo Y, Thomson RG, et al. Clinical features and natural history of progressive supranuclear palsy: a clinical cohort study. *Neurology.* 2003;60:910–916.

Nath U, Ben-Shlomo Y, Thomson RG, et al. The prevalence of PSP (Steele-Richardson-Olszewski syndrome) in the UK. *Brain.* 2001;124:1438–1449.

Newman GC. Treatment of progressive supranuclear palsy with tricyclic antidepressants. *Neurology.* 1985;35:1189–1193.

Nieforth KA, Golbe LI. Retrospective study of drug response in 87 patients with progressive supranuclear palsy. *Clin Neuropharmacol.* 1993;16:338–346.

Nigro S, Morelli M, Arabia G, et al. Magnetic resonance parkinsonism index and midbrain to pons ratio: which index better distinguishes progressive supranuclear palsy patients with a low degree of diagnostic certainty from patients with Parkinson disease? *Parkinsonism Relat Disord.* 2017;41:31–36.

Nuebling G, Hensler M, Paul S, et al. PROSPERA: a randomized, controlled trial evaluating rasagiline in progressive supranuclear palsy. *J Neurol.* 2016;263:1565–1574.

O'Sullivan SS, Massey LA, Williams DR, et al. Clinical outcomes of PSP and MSA. *Brain.* 2008;131:1362–1372.

Oba H, Yagishita A, Terada H, et al. New and reliable MRI diagnosis for progressive supranuclear palsy. *Neurology.* 2005;64:2050–2055.

Olszewski J, Steele J, Richardson JC. Pathological report on six cases of heterogeneous system degeneration. *J Neuropathol Exp Neurol.* 1963;23:187–188.

Osaki Y, Ben-Shlomo Y, Lees AJ, et al. Accuracy of clinical diagnosis of progressive supranuclear palsy. *Mov Disord.* 2004;19:181–189.

Osaki Y, Morita Y, Miyamoto Y, et al. Freezing of gait is an early clinical feature of progressive supranuclear palsy. *Neurol Clin Neurosci.* 2017;5:86–90.

Osaki Y, Wenning GK, Daniel SE, et al. Do published criteria improve clinical diagnostic accuracy in multiple system atrophy? *Neurology.* 2002;59:1486–1491.

Ou R, Song W, Wei Q, et al. Characteristics of nonmotor symptoms in progressive supranuclear palsy. *Parkinsons Dis.* 2016;2016:9730319.

Owens E, Krecke K, Ahlskog JE, et al. Highly specific radiographic marker predates clinical diagnosis in progressive supranuclear palsy. *Parkinsonism Relat Disord.* 2016;28:107–111.

Parkinson J. *An Essay on the Shaking Palsy.* Sherwood, Neely and Jones. London, 1817.

Passamonti L, Vázquez Rodríguez P, Hong YT, et al. ^{18}F-AV-1451 positron emission tomography in Alzheimer's disease and progressive supranuclear palsy. *Brain.* 2017;140:781–791.

Paviour DC, Thornton JS, Lees AJ, Jäger HR. Diffusion-weighted magnetic resonance imaging differentiates Parkinsonian variant of multiple-system atrophy from progressive supranuclear palsy. *Mov Disord.* 2007;22:68–74.

Pearce JM. Progressive supranuclear palsy (Steele-Richardson-Olszewski syndrome): a short historical review. *Neurologist.* 2007;13:302–304.

Pharr V, Uttl B, Stark M, et al. Comparison of apraxia in corticobasal degeneration and progressive supranuclear palsy. *Neurology.* 2001;56:957–963.

Picillo M, Erro R, Cuoco S, et al. MDS PSP criteria in real-life clinical setting: motor and cognitive characterization of subtypes. *Mov Disord.* 2018 Jul 8. doi: 10.1002/mds.27408.

Pillon B, Dubois B, Ploska A, et al. Severity and specificity of cognitive impairment in Alzheimer's, Huntington's, and Parkinson's diseases and progressive supranuclear palsy. *Neurology.* 1991;41:634–643.

Pollock NJ, Mirra SS, Binder LI, et al. Filamentous aggregates in Pick's disease, PSP, and Alzheimer's disease share antigenic determinants with microtubule-associated protein, tau. *Lancet.* 1986;2:1211.

Quattrone A, Nicoletti G, Messina D, et al. MR imaging index for differentiation of progressive supranuclear palsy from Parkinson disease and the Parkinson variant of multiple system atrophy. *Radiology.* 2008;246:214–221.

Rafal RD, Grimm RJ. Progressive supranuclear palsy: functional analysis of the response to methysergide and anti parkinsonian agents. *Neurology.* 1981;31:1507–1518.

Ramig LO, Sapir S, Fox C, et al. Changes in vocal loudness following intensive voice treatment (LSVT®) in individuals with Parkinson's disease: a comparison with untreated patients and normal age-matched controls. *Mov Dis.* 2001;16:79–83.

Respondek G, Kurz C, Arzberger T, et al. Which ante mortem clinical features predict progressive supranuclear palsy pathology? *Mov Disord.* 2017;32:995–1005.

Respondek G, Roeber S, Kretzschmar H, et al. Accuracy of the National Institute for Neurological Disorders and Stroke/Society for Progressive Supranuclear Palsy and neuroprotection and natural history in Parkinson plus syndromes criteria for the diagnosis of progressive supranuclear palsy. *Mov Disord.* 2013;28:504–509.

Respondek G, Stamelou M, Kurz C, et al; Movement Disorder Society–endorsed PSP Study Group. The phenotypic spectrum of progressive supranuclear palsy: a retrospective multicenter study of 100 definite cases. *Mov Disord.* 2014;29:1758–1766.

Richardson JC, Steele J, Olszewski J. Supranuclear ophthalmoplegia, pseudobulbar palsy, nuchal dystonia and dementia: a clinical report on eight cases of "heterogeneous system degeneration." *Transact Am Neurol Assoc.* 1963;88:25–29.

Robbins TW, James M, Owen AM, et al. Cognitive deficits in progressive supranuclear palsy, Parkinson's disease, and multiple system atrophy in tests sensitive to frontal lobe dysfunction. *J Neurol Neurosurg Psychiatry.* 1994;57:79–88.

Rojas JC, Bang J, Lobach IV, et al; AL-108-231 Investigators. CSF neurofilament light chain and phosphorylated tau 181 predict disease progression in PSP. *Neurology.* 2018;90:e273-e281.

Rojas JC, Karydas A, Bang J, et al. Plasma neurofilament light chain predicts progression in progressive supranuclear palsy. *Ann Clin Transl Neurol.* 2016;3:216–25.

Ros R, Gómez Garre P, Hirano M, et al. Genetic linkage of autosomal dominant progressive supranuclear palsy to 1q31.1. *Ann Neurol.* 2005;57:634–641.

Sale P, Castiglioni D, De Pandis MF, et al. The Lee Silverman Voice Treatment (LSVT®) speech therapy in progressive supranuclear palsy. *Eur J Phys Rehabil Med.* 2015; 51:569–574.

Salsano E, Umeh C, Rufa A, et al. Vertical supranuclear gaze palsy in Niemann-Pick type C disease. *Neurol Sci.* 2012;33:1225–1232.

Sanchez-Contreras MY, Kouri N, Cook CN, et al. Replication of progressive supranuclear palsy genome-wide association study identifies SLCO1A2 and DUSP10 as new susceptibility loci. *Mol Neurodegener.* 2018;13:37.

Santos-Santos MA, Mandelli ML, Binney RJ, et al. Features of patients with nonfluent/agrammatic primary progressive aphasia with underlying progressive supranuclear palsy pathology or corticobasal degeneration. *JAMA Neurol.* 2016; 73:733–742.

Schlesinger I, Klesier A, Yarnitsky D. Pain in progressive supranuclear palsy. *Clin Neuropharmacol.* 2009;32:163–164.

Schmotz C, Richinger C, Lorenzl S. High burden and depression among late-stage idiopathic Parkinson disease and progressive supranuclear palsy caregivers. *J Geriatr Psychiatry Neurol.* 2017;30:267–272.

Schonfeld SM, Golbe LI, Safer JN, et al. Computerized tomographic findings in progressive supranuclear palsy: correlation with clinical grade. *Mov Disord.* 1987;2:263–278.

Schonhaut DR, McMillan CT, Spina S, et al. ^{18}F-flortaucipir tau positron emission tomography distinguishes established progressive supranuclear palsy from controls and Parkinson disease: a multicenter study. *Ann Neurol.* 2017;82:622–634.

Schrag A, Ben-Shlomo Y, Quinn NP. Prevalence of progressive supranuclear palsy and multiple system atrophy: a cross-sectional study. *Lancet.* 1999;354:1771–1775.

Schrag A, Selai C, Davis J, et al. Health-related quality of life in patients with progressive supranuclear palsy. *Mov Disord.* 2003;18:1464–1469.

Schrag A, Selai C, Quinn N, et al. Measuring quality of life in PSP: the PSP-QoL. *Neurology.* 2006;67:39–44.

Sequeira AL-S, Rizzo J-R, Rucker JC. Clinical approach to supranuclear brainstem saccadic gaze palsies. *Front Neurol.* 2017;8:429.

Sonies BC. Speech and swallowing disturbances. In: Litvan I, Agid Y, eds. *Progressive Supranuclear Palsy: Clinical and Research Approaches.* New York, NY: Oxford University Press; 1992:240–253.

Stamelou M, Reuss A, Pilatus U, et al. Short-term effects of coenzyme Q10 in progressive supranuclear palsy: a randomized, placebo-controlled trial. *Mov Disord.* 2008;23:942–949.

Stamelou M, Schöpe J, Wagenpfeil S, et al. AL-108-231 Investigators, Tauros Investigators, and MDS-Endorsed PSP Study Group. Power calculations and placebo effect for future clinical trials in progressive supranuclear palsy. *Mov Disord.* 2016;31:742–747.

Steele JC, Richardson JC, Olszewski J. Progressive supranuclear palsy: a heterogeneous degeneration involving the brain stem, basal ganglia and cerebellum with vertical gaze and pseudobulbar palsy, nuchal dystonia and dementia. *Arch Neurol.* 1964;10:333–359.

Suteerawattananon M, MacNeill B, Protas EJ. Supported treadmill training for gait and balance in a patient with progressive supranuclear palsy. *Phys Ther.* 2002;82:485–495.

Tacik P, Sanchez-Contreras M, Rademakers R, et al. Genetic disorders with tau pathology: a review of the literature and report of two patients with tauopathy and positive family histories. *Neurodegener Dis.* 2016;16:12–21.

Tang CC, Poston KL, Eckert T, et al. Differential diagnosis of parkinsonism: a metabolic imaging study using pattern analysis. *Lancet Neurol.* 2010;9:149–158.

Tellez-Nagel I, Wisniewski HM. Ultrastructure of neurofibrillary tangles in Steele-Richardson-Olszewski syndrome. *Arch Neurol.*1973;29:324–327.

Tetrud JW, Golbe LI, Forno LS, et al. Autopsy-proven progressive supranuclear palsy in two siblings. *Neurology.* 1996;46:931–934.

Tolosa E, Litvan I, Höglinger GU, et al. A phase 2 trial of the GSK-3 inhibitor tideglusib in progressive supranuclear palsy. *Mov Disord.* 2014;29:470–478.

Tretiakoff KN. Contribution a l'Etude de L'Anatomie pathologique du Locus Niger de Soemmering avec quelques déductions relatives à la pathogénie des troubles du tonus musculaire et De La Maladie de Parkinson. MD dissertation, University of Paris, 1919.

Troost BT. Neuro-ophthalmological aspects. In: Litvan I, Agid Y, eds. *Progressive Supranuclear Palsy: Clinical and Research Approaches.* New York, NY: Oxford University Press; 1992:184–222.

Tsukamoto K, Matsusue E, Kanasaki Y, et al. Significance of apparent diffusion coefficient measurement for the differential diagnosis of multiple system atrophy, progressive supranuclear palsy, and Parkinson's disease: evaluation by 3.0-T MR imaging. *Neuroradiology.* 2012;54:947–955.

Uitti B, Santacruz P, Litvan I, et al. Caregiving in progressive supranuclear palsy. *Neurology.* 1998;51:1303–1309.

Vidal JS, Vidailhet M, Derkinderen P, et al. Risk factors for progressive supranuclear palsy: a case-control study in France. *J Neurol Neurosurg Psychiatry.* 2009;80:1271–1274.

Vizcarra JA, Lang AE, Sethi KD, et al. Vascular Parkinsonism: deconstructing a syndrome. *Mov Disord.* 2015;30:886–894.

Wakatsuki A, Tsujihata M, Miyake O, Ito H, Itatani H, Udaka F. Vesicourethral function study and application of urinary alarm in progressive supranuclear palsy [in Japanese]. *Hinyokika Kiyo.* 1993;39:891–897.

Walsh CM, Ruoff L, Walker K, et al. Sleepless night and day, the plight of progressive supranuclear palsy. *Sleep.* 2017;40. doi: 10.1093/sleep/zsx154.

Wani WY, Chatham JC, Darley-Usmar V, et al. O-GlcNAcylation and neurodegeneration. *Brain Res Bull.* 2017;133:80–87.

Warnecke T, Oelenberg S, Teismann I, et al. Endoscopic characteristics and levodopa responsiveness of swallowing function in progressive supranuclear palsy. *Mov Disord.* 2010;25: 1239–1245.

Weiner WJ, Minagar A, Shulman LM. Pramipexole in progressive supranuclear palsy. *Neurology.* 1999;52:873–874.

West T, Hu Y, Verghese PB, et al. Preclinical and clinical development of ABBV-8E12, a humanized anti-tau antibody, for treatment of Alzheimer's disease and other tauopathies. *J Prev Alzheimers Dis.* 2017:236–241.

Whitwell JL, Höglinger GU, Antonini A, et al; Movement Disorder Society–endorsed PSP Study Group. Radiological biomarkers for diagnosis in PSP: where are we and where do we need to be? *Mov Disord.* 2017;32:955–971.

Whitwell JL, Master AV, Avula R, et al. Clinical correlates of white matter tract degeneration in progressive supranuclear palsy. *Arch Neurol.* 2011;68:753–760.

Whitwell JL, Xu J, Mandrekar JN, et al. Rates of brain atrophy and clinical decline over 6 and 12-month intervals in PSP: determining sample size for treatment trials. *Parkinsonism Relat Disord.* 2012;18:252–256.

Wiblin L, Lee M, Burn D. Palliative care and its emerging role in multiple system atrophy and progressive supranuclear palsy. *Parkinsonism Relat Disord.* 2017;34:7–14.

Williams DR, de Silva R, Paviour DC, et al. Characteristics of two distinct clinical phenotypes in pathologically proven progressive supranuclear palsy: Richardson's syndrome and PSP-parkinsonism. *Brain.* 2005; 128(Pt 6):1247–1258.

Williams DR, Holton JL, Strand K, et al. Pure akinesia with gait freezing: a third clinical phenotype of progressive supranuclear palsy. *Mov Disord.* 2007;22:2235–2241.

Wittmann CW, Wszolek MF, Shulman JM, et al. Tauopathy in Drosophila: neurodegeneration without neurofibrillary tangles. *Science.*2001;293:711–714.

Yasui K, Inoue Y, Kanbayaski T, et al. CSF orexin levels of Parkinson's disease, dementia with Lewy bodies, progressive supranuclear palsy and corticobasal degeneration. *J Neurol Sci.* 2006;250:120–123.

Yoon WT, Chung EJ, Lee SH, et al. Clinical analysis of blepharospasm and apraxia of eyelid opening in patients with parkinsonism. *J Clin Neurol.* 2005;1:159–165.

Zadikoff C, Lang AE. Apraxia in movement disorders. *Brain.* 2005;128(Pt 7):1480–1497.

Zampieri C, Di Fabio RP. Balance and eye movement training to improve gait in people with progressive supranuclear palsy: quasi-randomized clinical trial. *Phys Ther.* 2008;88: 1460–1473.

Zampieri C, Di Fabio RP. Improvement of gaze control after balance and eye movement training in patients with progressive supranuclear palsy: a quasi-randomized controlled trial. *Arch Phys Med Rehabil.* 2009;90:263–270.

Zampieri C, Di Fabio RP. Progressive supranuclear palsy: disease profile and rehabilitation strategies. *Phys Ther.* 2006;86:870–880.

INDEX

Italic page numbers indicate tables and figures.

ABOUT THE AUTHOR

LAWRENCE I. GOLBE, MD, is emeritus professor of neurology at Rutgers Robert Wood Johnson Medical School in New Brunswick, New Jersey. He chairs the Scientific Advisory Board of CurePSP and serves as its clinical director. His research centers on the epidemiology, etiology, treatment, and clinimetrics of PSP and Parkinson disease.

Printed and bound by CPI Group (UK) Ltd, Croydon, CR0 4YY

16/04/2025

14658332-0005